THE HANDBOOK OF
SCHOOL ART THERAPY

ABOUT THE AUTHOR

Janet Bush, A.T.R.-BC, started art therapy as a pilot program in the Dade County Public Schools, Miami, Florida, and soon demonstrated the potential value of an art therapy approach. She is presently serving as Department Chairperson in the Division of Exceptional Student Education, where she directs a program with twenty master art therapists who provide services for over 400 emotionally disturbed Dade County students.

Ms. Bush began her career as an art educator, having received a B.A. degree in art from Ohio State University. Graduate art therapy studies at Hahnemann Medical University, in Philadelphia, led her to work in a public school setting and to spawn the idea of applying art therapy in the public schools.

Her model program for the public schools made a major contribution to the field of art therapy, and was recognized by the American Art Therapy Association. She subsequently received a Distinguished Service Award for her clinical work with children.

Ms. Bush is a registered, board certified, practicing clinical art psychotherapist, a founding member of the Florida Art Therapy Association, a university instructor, and a nationally known speaker and lecturer on art therapy in the schools. She has authored a number of articles, and has served as a consultant in many clinical and educational settings. In the Dade County Public Schools, she has successfully launched the first full art therapy program in a public school setting in the country, and her pioneering work has energized the practice of art therapy in public schools nationwide.

THE HANDBOOK OF SCHOOL ART THERAPY

Introducing Art Therapy Into A School System

By

JANET BUSH, A.T.R.-BC

Department Chairperson
Division of Exceptional Student Education
Dade County Public Schools
Miami, Florida

With a Foreword by

Myra F. Levick, PH.D., A.T.R.-BC, HLM

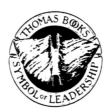

CHARLES C THOMAS • PUBLISHER, LTD.
Springfield • Illinois • U.S.A.

Published and Distributed Throughout the World by

CHARLES C THOMAS • PUBLISHER, LTD.
2600 South First Street
Springfield, Illinois 62794-9265

© *1997 by* CHARLES C THOMAS • PUBLISHER, LTD.
ISBN 0-398-06740-6 (cloth)
ISBN 0-398-06741-4 (paper)
Library of Congress Catalog Card Number: 96-48444

With THOMAS BOOKS *careful attention is given to all details of manufacturing
and design. It is the Publisher's desire to present books that are satisfactory as to
their physical qualities and artistic possibilities and appropriate for their particular
use.* THOMAS BOOKS *will be true to those laws of quality that assure a good
name and good will.*

Printed in the United States of America
SC-R-3

Library of Congress Cataloging-in-Publication Data

Bush, Janet.
   The handbook of school art therapy : introducing art therapy into
a school system / by Janet Bush ; with a foreword by Myra F. Levick.
     p.   cm.
   Includes bibliographical references and index.
   ISBN 0-398-06740-6 (cloth). — ISBN 0-398-06741-4 (pbk.)
   1. Art therapy for children. 2. School psychology. I. Title.
RJ505.A7B87   1997
615.8'5156'083—dc21   96-48444
                                               CIP

CONTRIBUTORS

SARAH P. HITE, M.S., M.S.ED., A.T.R.–BC
Graduate Art Therapy Program
Eastern Virginia Medical School
Norfolk, Virginia

JENNIFER LOMBROIA, M.A., A.T.R.
Clinical Art Therapist
Dade County Public Schools
Miami, Florida

LINDA JO PFEIFFER, ED.D., A.T.R.
Clinical Art Therapist
Dade County Public Schools
Miami, Florida

In memory of my parents
Louis and Elva Bush

FOREWORD

This book transcends the concept evoked by the term "handbook." It is a comprehensive work describing the day-to-day, hands-on experience of Janet Bush as she struggled to bring art therapy into the public school system.

The outline of her image begins to emerge in the Preface and Introduction. She rightly points out that the traditional purpose of schools was to teach children knowledge. And if they did not learn, it was not within the province of the educator in the school system to deal with the matter.

As an art educator, Ms. Bush, like so many others, began to recognize the indicators of cognitive and emotional problems surfacing in the artwork of some of her students. She describes how this growing awareness led to her initial interest in art therapy and how it became the catalyst for forging the new frontier. She carefully pursued a graduate degree in art therapy, at that time, a nascent field. Innovatively, she tested her inclination by requesting clinical placement in a public school setting, then based her thesis on her experience: She focused on being available to work with children who could not remain in the classroom. Armed with the success and the confidence she had gained, she methodically set the stage for what would become years of an uphill battle.

In the very first chapter, Ms. Bush succinctly lays out the rationale for introducing art therapy into the school system, then spells out the delivery of art therapy services as she encompasses consultation, assessment and intervention, professional development, research, and program planning and evaluation. She makes a cogent point that the addition of a registered art therapist within the school setting is critical to the fulfillment of the federal mandate, passed in 1975, to mainstream all disabled children.

Her history of art therapy in the schools is well documented and serves as a basis for further appreciation of this book. There was only one other program in the country when Ms. Bush proposed her pilot program to introduce art therapy into the Dade County Public School System. She describes her proposal, its implementation, and the response from school administrators and faculty at its completion. New doors were opened and her work continued.

She helps the reader to understand the many facets of her self-determined task. Ms. Bush makes it very clear that as the structure and needs of education shift and change, the art therapist must be prepared to meet the challenges and must work to become an integral part of the education of our children, in conjunction, both, with their cognitive and emotional parameters.

In detailing her own progression in the development of the Art Therapy Program at the Dade County Public School System, she covers every aspect of the utilization of art therapy and the role of art therapists in the school. Her comprehensive discussion and her evaluation of the pilot program are extremely useful for art therapists, teachers, and parents. They can serve as a guide to understanding the many problems inherent in introducing a new approach to a traditional setting. For those who would replicate her model, she offers her experience and the hard-earned knowledge she has acquired through such intervening areas as hiring art therapists, the physical environment, public relations, and strategies for funding.

Ms. Bush started as an army of one, fought a battle, and clearly emerged the victor. There are now 20 art therapists employed in the art therapy program she directs. But it is obvious that she is not satisfied. She challenges art therapists, school teachers, administrators, and parents to share in the effort. There is a legitimate inducement for joining her team as she points to the speed with which the world moves forward, and the snail's pace at which traditional educational settings proceed, which makes them appear to be standing still. There is also a challenge to educators of art teachers and art therapists. She correctly points out the paucity of trained specialists, and emphasizes the fact that trained specialists are needed to serve the growing numbers of identified populations with special needs.

The art therapy program directed by Ms. Bush in the Dade County Public School System is the only one of its kind—and it is a model for the country. She has indeed provided a "handbook" of information for teachers sensitive to their students' needs, parents concerned about their children, art therapists who want to work in a school system, and educators who guide teachers and art therapists. I am sure they will all want to keep the knowledge she has been able to amass close at hand.

MYRA F. LEVICK

PREFACE

This volume is a handbook for clinicians and educators, and for concerned parents everywhere who are seeking nontraditional intervention methods for the thousands of children and adolescents who need to overcome emotional interference with their cognitive and emotional progress. The physical, organic, developmental, environmental, social, and emotional conditions that afflict students have not been effectively countered heretofore because the traditional methods of verbal counseling and assessment have not met their total needs. Art therapy is a nontraditional intervention method designed to bridge the gap between the information acquired about children by educators and the observations made about children's problems by such school clinicians as counselors and psychologists.

Educators apply cognitive standards to help children reach their academic potential. They do not normally assist children with mental health intervention. Counselors assist children in the area of mental health, but with a verbal modality. School psychologists are generally involved with the testing and placement of children who have special needs. The art therapist relates to all of these professionals and their tailored intervention methods and to all of these children, then seeks, by a combined verbal and visual approach and the application of diagnostic and prescriptive methods, to access the inner feelings of the children. The children reveal their personal worries to the art therapist through their artwork. The art therapist is able to assess their emotional damage and to institute remediation measures. With one approach, an art therapist can capture both the cognitive and emotional responses of a student, and can produce the feedback sought by a school treatment team.

This handbook on school art therapy stems from the years of work conducted by the School Art Therapy Program of the Dade County Public Schools, Miami, Florida, where art therapy services have been a regular part of the educational program for students since 1979. The program is funded through monies appropriated for exceptional students.

The handbook provides a comprehensive treatment of the body of knowledge on which art therapy was founded and on which it continues to grow and will perhaps shape the future profession. It is intended as a single source of information on the profession's current challenges. Chapters range from discussions on theory and development to discussions on the nuts and bolts of daily practice. The hope is that it will become a major reference work which practicing art therapists, educators, and school mental health personnel can consult for practical suggestions.

If this handbook has a major theme, it is that the profession of art therapy has evolved to encompass a wide range of applications. Although the specialty was traditionally a part of medical intervention for psychiatric patients, its horizons have expanded. In school settings, it has dealt with the so-called normal youngster, with the disabled youngster, and with the youngster experiencing emotional problems. The handbook reflects the growing sophistication of the profession of art therapy and its interface with other fields—particularly, the education field. Art therapy in the schools represents new ideas, healthy controversy, and fresh challenges.

The book is divided into sixteen chapters, each devoted to a major facet of the practice of art therapy in a school setting. The material will no doubt be revised in the years to come because the practice of art therapy is in a state of evolution, and its application to school settings will continue to change as refined approaches replace old ideas. Perhaps some day there will be art therapists in every school, public and private, in which case, traditional education will have been enriched by the need to suit the times.

The completion of this handbook would not have been possible without the wide-ranging encouragement I have received from many people. I want to thank my friend Lori La Medica for her patience, support, and objective review; chapter contributors, Sarah Hite, Jennifer Lombroia, and Linda Jo Pfeiffer, each of whom offered knowledge, ideas, and fresh approaches; and Don Jones and Myra Levick, who provided me with the requisite training needed to work successfully in this field—they encouraged my dreams, taught me the body of knowledge needed to achieve success, and led me to continually ask questions. Myra Levick has also served as my consultant and mentor through the years, providing me with invaluable support and reinforcing my professional capabilities. Her pioneering work in the field of art therapy has been a solid foundation for the work I have undertaken. I acknowledge, too, the help of Sylvia Shubert, who has worked with me to put this material in final form; and of Will Gordillo, Director, Ronald Felton, Executive Director, and Terri Reynolds, Assistant Superintendent, Office of Exceptional Student Education, Dade County Public Schools, who have contributed in large measure to the growth of art therapy in the Miami public school district through their recognition of its value in the lives of a considerable number of children. In conclusion, I cannot fail to express my appreciation to the person in the Dade County Public School System who encouraged me to introduce art therapy in the schools and to continue its implementation—Jacqueline Hinchey-Sipes— whose foresight and dedication to all children enabled art therapy to find a place in the Dade County public schools; and to the many art therapists who have worked with me through the years in Dade County and elsewhere, who believe, as I do, that children deserve the best. My parents would have appreciated my contribution to the profession of art therapy, and I embrace their memory as a guiding light in my work.

I will always appreciate the peace and serenity I experienced while writing this book on the enchanting island of Nantucket, Massachusetts.

Although this book is related to my work in the Dade County Public Schools, I have written it in my private capacity. I do not claim official support or endorsement from the Dade County Public Schools or from the State of Florida Department of Education

JANET BUSH

INTRODUCTION

I had lunch with a former staff member who was visiting from out of town. Over sandwiches, we updated each other on our lives. It was not long before the topic of art therapy came up. Maryann was living in a small Florida town where she was working as an art teacher in three public school settings. Even though she is a registered art therapist, she could not perform art therapy services in her schools because public schools were not funded for such work.

Obviously, the town and its public schools saw meeting conventional education standards as their priority. Maryann had the necessary credentials to work as an art teacher. The State of Florida Art Education teaching certification she held guaranteed her eligibility for art instruction. Maryann was hired to teach 25 art classes a week.

Although Maryann had been able to get her foot in the door of the town's public schools, she had not been able to do much more than wiggle her toes. She had spent three long years pursuing public relations activities and inservice education programs with the thought of promoting interest in art therapy. She was now intent on finding other means of establishing art therapy in her school district.

We discussed various funding strategies and ways to implement services, and I believe Maryann left our luncheon with a bit more confidence and enthusiasm than she had arrived with. She knew that what I had suggested was possible, since when I came to the Dade County Public Schools as a registered art therapist with an art education background, in 1976, school personnel had no idea what the potential for art therapy was. Yet today, there are twenty full-time art therapists employed in over 28 Dade County public schools. The strategies I had offered Maryann were based on the tried-and-true techniques implemented in the Dade County school district through the years.

This book has been designed to help individuals like Maryann introduce the principles of art therapy and implement the techniques needed in school settings, but with the understanding and caution that art therapy in the schools is in the process of "blazing" its trail. It should not be used as art education in an academic sense, nor should it serve as a substitute for counseling or school psychological services. Each field is a separate entity, and has a valid radius of operation. The fields are not interchangeable and are inadequate as replacements for each other. Art therapy utilizes philosophical bases and selected strategies from the other disciplines to extract innermost expressions from students, but its express purpose is to induce results that are compatible with its specialized corrective mission. Youngsters with special needs may, in fact, need to have all of the services offered—art therapy, art education for academic purposes, counseling, and school psychological services.

When holding on to a rip cord, a fall back position carries a price. The need is to go forward, to pull the rip cord, and to engage in a free fall to a tried though new form of learning. Countless numbers of children have gone unassisted through the years because art therapy was not in a position to pull the rip cord. I believe we have now managed to reach a significant moment of change, and that in the future we will be able to benefit all children in school through the establishment of art therapy as a specialized, unalloyed support service.

CONTENTS

LIST OF ILLUSTRATIONS

Case of John Franklin

THE HANDBOOK OF
SCHOOL ART THERAPY

Chapter 1

RATIONALE FOR THE INTRODUCTION OF ART THERAPY IN SCHOOLS

Art therapy was traditionally the province of hospitals and mental health centers. The Dade County Public Schools recognized the strengths and advantages that could accrue from the use of art therapy to stem a variety of unacceptable behaviors. In its consistent effort to put students with problems on the right path in their studies, it introduced a pilot art therapy program in the 1979–80 school year.

It has since confirmed that art therapists are unique in the work they perform with students because they combine the attention they give to the verbal communications of the students with the special attention they pay to the nonverbal communications of the students, and they personalize their contact with the students. They are specially equipped to explore the personal problems of the children and the potential revealed by individual children, and then to develop pathways for learning that are not feasible with traditional methods of instruction. Art therapists are qualified to observe and analyze behavior, art products, and student communications, to make diagnostic assessments, and to formulate treatment plans that provide total art therapy coverage. They are not only prepared to deal with the students assigned to them as part of their regular workload, they are capable of taking on random diagnostic work and treatment when called upon to assess students referred to them from a variety of districtwide programs. They are, in addition, qualified to conduct inservice workshops for art and exceptional education teachers, and for psychologists, counselors, and administrators.

Art therapists utilize art products and individual associations with art products to help generate physical, emotional, and learning skills that can foster compatible relationships between students and their inner and outer worlds. Students in art therapy who come to an improved understanding of their problems may even be helped, through art

3

experiences, to resolve their problems. By gaining new understanding of themselves, they learn to face their conflicts.

An apt analogy might picture them as facing life as they would face a blank art canvas: seizing the opportunity to rework maladjusted patterns into creative adaptive patterns. By likening themselves to artists who can repaint canvasses they do not like after the paint is dry, they can, in a sense, learn to paint over their problems to attain new solutions. The way they face the canvas can become a metaphor for the way they face life.

√ COMPREHENSIVE SCHOOL ART THERAPY
SERVICES DELIVERY

The duties of school art therapists are as broad as the ensuing description is long: School art therapists provide a range of services for students, direct and indirect, which require involvement with the entire educational system—students, teachers, administrators, and other school personnel; families, surrogate caretakers, community and regional agencies; resources that support the educational process; the organizational, physical, temporal, and curricular variables that play major roles within the system; and a variety of other factors that may be important on an individual basis. The intent of these services is to promote mental health and to facilitate learning.

Comprehensive school art therapy activities complement one another, and are therefore most accurately viewed as an integrated and coordinated whole rather than as discrete services. However, to promote an indepth understanding of them, I have listed and described them separately under the following categories:

Consultation

- Collaboration on mental health and behavioral and educational concerns is recurrent with school personnel, and with parents and outside people when consultation is merited.
- Inservice and other skill enhancement activities are provided for school personnel, for parents, and for others in the community on learning, development, and behavior.
- Collaborative relationships are developed with the students themselves to involve them in the assessment, intervention, and program evaluation procedures.

Assessment

- Assessment practices are utilized that increase the likelihood of effective educational intervention and followup.
- Assessment reports become a permanent part of a student's records.
- The assessment instruments used have established reliability and validity for the intended purpose and population.
- Nonbiased assessment techniques help to maximize student achievement and educational success.

Intervention

- Direct and indirect interventions are provided to help the students function.
- Programs are designed to enhance cognitive, emotional, social, and vocational development.
- Assistance is given to school personnel, to personnel at community agencies, and to parents, consisting of, but not limited to, inservice training, organization, development, program planning and evaluation, parent counseling, and parent education.

Professional Training and Development

- Professional training and development are accomplished by means of a continuing professional development program. Release time and financial support to cover meeting fees are provided by the school or school district.
- Peer review is incorporated for mutual assistance and self-examination.
- The supervision of all school art therapists is sufficient to ensure accountable services.
- A coordinated plan for accountability and evaluation of all services is implemented and revised as needed.

Research

- School art therapists design, conduct, and document their own research. They also make use of the general body of professional research. Both the applied and the basic research focus on the psychological and artistic functioning of human beings, on art therapy assessment tools and procedures, and on art therapy treatment and techniques.

- Research ranges from engaging in support or advisory services to taking direct responsibility for one or more major components of a project. Components may involve planning, data collection, data analysis, dissemination, or the translation of the knowledge acquired into practical applications within the school community.

Program Planning and Evaluation

- The school art therapists serve on committees that are responsible for planning and developing educational and educationally related activities.
- The planning and evaluation of art therapy services assist in decision-making activities.

The process leads to a variety of fortuitous results. It can, for example, help to identify problems; lead to solutions to problems; divert unproductive behavior to healthy expression; control unhealthy impulses; and reduce feelings of guilt. Ventilating explosive feelings can untether enough energy to develop good relations with others, and to form lasting friendships. It can help students to find themselves—to know who and what they are. Needless to say, the many new outlets opened to the students can trigger the kind of corrective emotion that generates self-growth. With the insights gained from treatment, they can eventually cope with their lives and with life.

The 1975 federal mandate, Public Law 94-142, The Education for All Handicapped Children Act, and the Individuals with Disabilities Act (IDEA), Public Law 101-476, which is the reauthorization bill for P.L. 94-142, deal with children who have disabilities. They include youngsters who are mentally retarded, hearing impaired, speech or language impaired, visually impaired, seriously emotionally disturbed, orthopedically impaired, and autistic, and youngsters who have traumatic brain injury, other health impairments, and specific learning disabilities.

Individuals recognized as disabled are entitled to receive special educational and related services. The Senate Report on the Code of Regulations for Public Law 94-142 clearly defines art therapy as a related service that can assist a disabled child to benefit from education (Section 121a.305). However, efforts should be made not only to strengthen the program for recognized disabled students, but for students who have not been identified as disabled and who would profit equally from art therapy treatment—children who experience difficulty at school as a result of social or emotional problems stemming from such sources as a crisis at home, the death of a significant person, parental separation or divorce, or abuse. Art therapy is equipped to offer a therapeutic/ diagnostic/prescriptive approach both to students who have been identified as disabled and to students who may not qualify for exceptional student programs but who have special needs. Furthermore, many students who are not well served by traditional counseling can profit from the graphic avenues of communication found in art therapy. Art therapy helps them to reconcile their emotional conflicts and leads them toward self-awareness and personal growth (AATA, 1986). Art therapy is, in effect, a catalyst that takes students with varying special needs and, through art, helps them to improve their outlook on life.

Chapter 2

THE DEVELOPMENT OF
SCHOOL ART THERAPY

School art therapy is a recent phenomenon. Documented scientific facts have never been turned up to substantiate earlier development. The closest approximation to a verifiable chronological history is the largely anecdotal series of reports prepared by the Dade County Public Schools in conjunction with the program it has had in operation since the 1979–80 school year. Although the Miami, Florida, school district is only the fourth largest in the country, it is the first educational entity to have perceived the advantages of **comprehensive** art therapy services. Its current program is well established, and the belief is that in time the program will be expanded to serve all categories of students.

Art therapy in Dade County began as an extension of the Dade County Art Education program. Other school art therapy programs started in the United States appear to have developed differently.

Under the Department of Exceptional Student Education, Felice W. Cohen had introduced art therapy to a Texas school district as early as 1975 (Art Psychotherapy, pp. 121–135). The services were designed to provide research on the possibility of utilizing art therapy as a diagnostic, screening, and therapeutic tool within a behavior modification model. As no job description or salary rating was provided, the art therapist was hired as a part-time consultant. Since there was no departmental classification for an art therapist, it was not known which meetings and workshops the art therapist should attend. The study identified the need to follow protocol with school administrators, and to keep appropriate personnel informed in order to develop rapport and to accomplish necessary tasks. Education of faculty and staff was identified to assist the teaching staff in understanding both the art therapy procedures and the individual students. However, this project was funded for six to eight months only, and there were no reliable and valid conclusions drawn. Empirical reports did document the benefits associated with the use of art therapy in the schools for diagnostic and screening purposes, and it was the author's judgment that art therapy should be used to personalize both the educational and mental health needs of all children.

In West Allis, Wisconsin, the services emerged from special education. There, school art therapists received training in art therapy, in exceptional student education, and in art education. An art therapist also served as a resource person, making remedial art techniques available to classroom teachers through inservice training and individual consultation. Virginia Minar is credited as the first person to have concluded a long-term (three-year) pilot study of art therapy in the West Allis public schools in June 1977. The study was sponsored by the West Allis, Wisconsin School District. The study attested to the value of art therapy and the art experience as a remedial procedure that extends beyond the corrective treatment area into the preventive area.

Elsewhere, individuals who were professionally credentialed art therapists seem to have worked independently, on a continual basis, with both public and private school children. A number of them were in local art, special education, or mental health programs that were carried out under contractual agreements with State, community education or mental health agencies, or with private agencies that provided art therapy treatment and diagnostic and assessment services. Many of them worked with both nondisabled and disabled children in therapeutic art programs, for example, Cohen (1974), Pine (1974), Anderson (1978, 1992), Fischer et al. (1978), and Stoner (1978). In addition, many art educators introduced the therapeutic aspects of art to nondisabled children in school art programs, for example, Cole (1941, 1966), Cane (1951), Lowenfeld (1957, 1970, 1975, 1987), and Robertson (1963).

Although originally founded within the context of art education, the Dade County Public Schools art therapy program moved out of the art education realm in the 1980s, and currently has twenty art therapists providing diagnostic and treatment services for youngsters in exceptional student education who have been identified as severely emotionally disturbed.

I chose to describe the present Dade County Public Schools model in detail in this book and to recommend it as a model for individuals and groups searching for guidelines to establish their own art therapy programs and services. Initially, since the State of Florida certified individuals as art teachers when they met the requirements for art education instruction, art therapists had to meet the requirements called for under art education regulations. Art therapists in the Dade County Public Schools can now maintain a state educator's certificate in any educational area. They must, however, have met the art therapy qualifications established by the American Art Therapy Association (AATA).

LEGISLATIVE INTENT

A healthy learning environment is essential to the educational process and to the general welfare of a school population. Various committees and legislative-related groups have established the fact that art therapy in the schools is conducive to the general welfare of the school population.

The Rockefeller panel (1977) was composed of twenty-five members who focused on the significance of the arts for American education. In the book *Coming To Our Senses* (Quin & Hanks, 1977), which resulted from the panel's study, reference was made to "convincing statistics" which demonstrated that meaningful artistic activities promoted clear gains in performance; for example, meaningful art programming had considerable influence on discipline and motivation.

The Senate and House Report (No. 96-712, May 15, 1980) on the Mental Health Systems Act of 1980 gave special attention to the creative arts therapies in the treatment of persons who required mental health services but who did not respond to traditional therapeutic modalities. The report acknowledged that such individuals had often been unserved or underserved because of obstacles to the establishment and broader utilization of the arts therapies within mental health settings.

Through its governmental liaison representative, the American Art Therapy Association submitted testimony (LACAT, September 1982) to the U.S. Department of Education regarding P.L. 94-142 (known as IDEA after it was updated in 1990). This testimony cited exemplary art therapy programs both in public and private schools.

Standing for Individuals with Disabilities Education Act, IDEA (P.L. 101-476, 1990) is now the federal law that governs special education. IDEA orders school systems to create programs for children with specific problems. The law identifies different disabilities and helps determine how children will be classified and educated. Some youngsters have behavioral or emotional problems so profound, they can only be schooled in special centers staffed by teachers and mental health personnel. Other youngsters have medical needs and require nursing care. There are children with hearing and vision problems, and youngsters so sick they have to be taught in their homes or in hospital rooms.

In its original form, as P.L. 94-142, passed in 1975, IDEA had identified art therapy as a viable service that may benefit a child who requires special education. This made it possible for school systems to allocate monies to help fund art therapy. Every school district now receives extra funding when disabled students are identified and served.

IMPACT OF ORGANIZATIONS

Art therapy gained slow and steady progress across the country, and as disabled children were mainstreamed into art classrooms on a more consistent basis, the awareness that art therapists could serve as professional resource consultants and service providers took on importance. The recognition led to a joint conference on August 7–8, 1980, conducted by the National Art Education Association and the American Art Therapy Association, under the sponsorship and funding of the National Committee on Arts for the Handicapped. It was the first attempt to assemble individuals in both fields to discuss and explore the role of art therapy in schools. The primary aim of the conference was to examine the mutual roles of art education and art therapy in providing art experiences for students with special needs (Bush, 1980). The conference program focused on the art teacher's role in a special education setting and in mainstreaming, and on the art therapist's role in clinical and educational settings. The conference was a milestone for art therapy in schools, as it solidified the professional standing of art therapists in schools and the training needs of art teachers in serving disabled students. Individual art therapists and art educators nationally known for their work in their respective fields attended the conference (Proceedings of the Joint Study Conference of the American Art Therapy Association and the National Committee on Arts for the Handicapped, 1980).

In 1985, The American Art Therapy Association published an official position statement, "Art Therapy in the Schools—A Position Paper of the American Art Therapy Association," relative to the questions raised at the study conference. It was intended for the use of such individuals and groups responsible for school art therapy programs in the United States as art therapists, school board members, administrators, supervisors, and any others interested in the application of art therapy in the schools. The position paper documented the purposes, principles, and standards for school art therapy programs. It reflected the official position of the Association, which was directed toward the promotion and recognition of educationally sound art therapy programs in the United States.

As a followup to the position statement, the Association's subcommittee and contributing art therapists and school administrators developed an accompanying resource packet that included sample job descriptions, goals, objectives, referral forms, and other useful guidelines for art therapists working in schools (American Art Therapy Association, 1986). This packet is available from The American Art Therapy Association, and is recommended to individuals and groups seeking assistance and support for establishing art therapy services.

The Association is currently editing a list of standards of practice for school art therapists that will assist individuals and groups in formulating new programs and in strengthening old programs (Bush, 1993).

MAJOR ISSUE IN THE DEVELOPMENT
OF SCHOOL ART THERAPY

Historically, school art therapy grew out of a specific need in school systems for the identification and remediation of students with learning problems. School children also had an array of behavioral problems that were associated with the learning process.

Art therapy can help children whose behavioral processes go awry. Nevertheless, the literature describing university training programs not only fails to include courses that are specific to the practice of school art therapy, but omits the linking of school art therapy to existing comprehensive fields of allied study. Some universities do provide training in **clinical approaches.** Labeled psychoanalytically-oriented art therapy, developmental art therapy, adaptive art therapy, and cognitive-behavioral art therapy, this multiplicity of training approaches for psychiatric settings prepares art therapists for traditional clinically-oriented practices. There is no bridge, in the use of these practices, to a school environment. University training, therefore, does not offer a unified track of specialization for prospective art therapists who want to work in schools. Furthermore, the undergraduate core curriculum is too generalized to prepare students for the field of art therapy, although it can prepare them to work as aides. Specialization needed to work as an art therapist can only be obtained on a graduate level, but since current graduate level courses of study are primarily focused on the practice of art therapy in clinical settings, the course work and internship for educational settings has yet to be developed.

Specialized graduate course work in school art therapy would create substantive job knowledge and opportunities. It would prepare individuals to make the transition from a professional clinical environment to an educational environment. It would also allow for a distinct separation in careers by providing the opportunity to place the emphasis either on a clinical approach or on a school approach. Furthermore, it would trigger action by state departments of education in the area of certification.

A small step has been taken to deal with the problem. Some schools, such as Eastern Virginia Medical School, in Norfolk, Virginia (Course Catalog, 1994) and Ursuline College, in Cleveland, Ohio (Course Catalog, 1994), offer elective courses—not an entire program.

In the breach, a student-patient population exists, waiting for services that are not available, and a potential school art therapy professional population cannot move into the forefront fully prepared to provide the services. Worse still, the field of art therapy not only lacks a consistent training curriculum; it has never developed a consistent philosophical approach (Levick, 1989). The time has come not only for students to be given the opportunity to specialize in the area of school art therapy, but to be able to acquire a body of knowledge that will help them to come to equivalent or parallel conclusions and judgments.

Preparation should be equivalent to the preparation experienced by medical personnel in their specialized fields. A basic core curriculum should focus on the clinical application of art therapy—using art therapy as psychotherapy. Specialized tracks should lead from the core curriculum and should include such areas of study as school art therapy, medical art therapy, child/adolescent art therapy, family art therapy, art therapy for assessment and evaluation, art therapy research, and the use of art therapy for self-expression and appreciation. Other tracks should be opened as needed.

Although school art therapy has had to struggle to evolve its identity, the intensity of the ideal remains strong. Unfortunately, progress continues to limp along. With the possibilities inherent in such a viable field of endeavor, there is no acceptable excuse for a gap to exist between the availability of professional art therapy services in the school setting and the demonstrated need for the services. We must eliminate the counterproductive wait public agencies, parents, children, and other potential beneficiaries of school art therapy services now experience before they can profit from the advantages that accrue from this proven form of treatment.

The time has come to speed up our efforts and to organize a practical school implementation model that will help to insure the mental health of our youth, and to create an appropriate definition of a school art therapist, as well as to induce both the undergraduate and the graduate schools to prepare enough school art therapists who can guide our students to succeed. The twenty-first century is almost here. We must be prepared to thrive in it!

Chapter 3

LOOKING AT THE EDUCATION PICTURE

Our schools face unprecedented challenges. There are momentous changes underway in the nation. Our entire society is struggling to cope with massive technological advance, worldwide political upheaval, and an array of economic and social issues.

The composition of our school population has changed dramatically. Our people look to the schools to make the necessary adjustments and to lead the way into the twenty-first century. Our schools are expected to educate children who are poorer, who are more ethnically and linguistically diverse, and who have more individual handicaps than any group of students that has preceded them. Our schools are urged to prepare these students for a future that has not yet been invented, in a world that is being continually altered. The emergence of an information society, accelerated by technological innovation, has rendered the previously accepted and successful curriculum increasingly useless and hopelessly out of date. The "old" ways no longer work. Simply stated, the world has been changing more rapidly than have our schools. Although our educational system has been performing at or above the levels it has in the past, it has not kept pace with the intellectual, social, and emotional needs of our world, which have expanded significantly.

Resources are limited; needs are not. Notwithstanding, it is taken for granted that our nation's school system will meet all the challenges thrown its way, then emerge from the struggle with exemplary educational methods in place that represent excellence at every level. Such a feat cannot be accomplished without a suitable rise in the supply and expenditure of educational capital, nor without the most dedicated efforts of our student body. There are no resources to waste; each dollar spent on education must be targeted on what and who will return the most profit.

Business communities and the public are demanding that our schools become more "customer focused." But consider our customers! Even those who succeed in school and who score well on conventional tests have not been educated sufficiently well to cope successfully with the concatenation of growing demands—personal, vocational, and civic—in contemporary society. If the schools do not prepare more of our students for what lies ahead, they will be perceived to have failed.

Traditional educational values and well-established programs are coming under intense scrutiny. The push for accountability, as measured by student performance outcomes, is increasing. Educators must be prepared to ensure that educational achievement by all students, which will have a profound influence on the quality of life of the entire population for generations to come, is a realistic expectation. The greatest challenge facing educators is the need to prove to the American public that the education system can respond to the pressures in a positive way, that it can improve performance in the schools, and that it can have a telling impact on the future success of the children served by the schools. It is time to join forces to bring about the regeneration so sorely needed throughout our educational system. Our failure to make the changes that we need will have an adverse effect on the entire nation.

Art therapists can help to meet the challenge of the twenty-first century by upgrading programs designed to assist youngsters at risk in their climb toward academic and emotional reconstruction. When used for diagnostic and screening purposes, art therapy procedures can identify the youngsters at risk. When used for treatment, art therapy can help the youngsters to better understand themselves and how they function as individuals and as part of a family or group system. Art expression, spurred by the aims of art therapy, lends itself well to analysis and, as a result, to individual adjustment to life.

Art therapy in a school setting can offer children the opportunity to work through obstacles that are impeding their educational progress. It can facilitate appropriate social behavior and promote healthy affective development. It can maximize social and academic potential by leading the children to become more receptive to academic involvement.

In recent years there has been a growing awareness of the lift art therapy gives to educational endeavor. Sporadic progress has been made across the country in the schools that have implemented art therapy services. It is time to introduce art therapy programs in all schools nationwide if general student academic progress is to be insured.

Chapter 4

DEVELOPMENT OF ART THERAPY
IN THE DADE COUNTY PUBLIC SCHOOLS

PART ONE—THE PILOT PROGRAM

Dade County's Art Therapy Program developed from a one-year pilot model, a collaborative effort between various administrative offices in the Division of Elementary and Secondary Education and the Division of Exceptional Student Education. Implemented during the 1979–80 school year, the pilot program provided for a registered art therapist who also had art education certification. The program combined both art education objectives and art therapy objectives for selected disabled students in self-contained classrooms, and a staff development program for personnel who were interested in acquiring techniques and strategies for teaching art to mainstreamed disabled students. Emphasis was placed on the potential for replication of the pilot model and on the uniqueness of a combined art education and art therapy service for severely disabled students (Bush, 1979).

The combined art education and art therapy service was considered distinctive because it had originated within the art education department, and funding was available through the local monies for art education so long as the model helped address art education needs. The philosophy behind the approach was that it was based on sound theoretical and philosophical constructs, and that both fields would benefit from the mutual endeavor. Ms. Jacqueline Hinchey-Sipes, the Art Education Supervisor at the time, had recognized the possibilities inherent in a combined approach, and had educated school officials to the merits of such a project. Funding covered the personnel cost of one art therapist, and the cost of materials and supplies used during the pilot program.

The purpose of the program was to help serve the needs of severely disabled students who were presenting problems to art teachers. Such students needed specialized approaches and strategies if they were to be taught effectively, but the art teachers were not adequately trained to work with disabled populations that could not function in typical mainstreamed class situations.

I was the pilot program art therapist responsible both for teaching art education and providing art therapy services to severely disabled students. I held a State of Florida educator's certificate in art education and a master's degree in art therapy together with an art therapy credential, A.T.R. (Art Therapist Registered). This gave me the essentials needed to accommodate art education and art therapy to the differences presented by a range of students. Most of the art teachers lacked such combined credentials.

The pilot program consisted of three phases—Planning, Development, and Implementation.

Planning and Development

1. Administrative Planning Meetings

Initial approval of the 1979–80 Pilot Program was obtained by means of joint meetings attended by the Director for Exceptional Student Education, the Director of Elementary and Secondary Education, and the Supervisor for Art Education.

The Supervisor for Art Education and I held advisory meetings with the District Area Superintendents and their staffs. The meetings included discussions on the schools, classes, and exceptionalities that were to be served, as well as on the proposed staff development module that would be implemented during the school year. I then held meetings with school site principals on procedural plans. It is important to note that the Art Therapy Program was not just one person's undertaking; it was a system-wide pilot plan. Many meetings were held both prior to program implementation and during the pilot year. Input was solicited from all the administrators. I learned later that these meetings doubled as public relations strategies, because they gave officials an opportunity to "buy into" the program plans.

2. Reporting Procedures

Reporting procedures were developed during the planning phase, to provide for documentation of the pilot stage. Several forms were prepared. Included were a teacher visitation observation checklist, session/lesson plans, and summaries of teacher conferences and staff development sessions.

3. School Visitations

As the art therapist, I visited sixteen self-contained art classes in the elementary schools. The visitations gave me an opportunity to observe the abilities of disabled students, student-teacher relationships, and art teacher approaches to working with exceptional youngsters. The visitations made it possible, in part, to determine the content areas that would be dealt with in the proposed staff development program and to decide which exceptionalities should finally be selected for receipt of the art education therapist's services in the Pilot Program.

4. Identification of the Pilot Groups

All of the four school administrative areas in Dade County were included in the pilot program. One school was chosen in each administrative area. A different exceptionality was identified in each of the four schools. The identified schools and the rationale for selecting each school may be seen below.

ADMINIS-TRATIVE AREA	SCHOOL	EXCEPTION-ALITY	RATIONALE
North	Biscayne Gardens Elementary	Physically Impaired	The school had a large exceptional student education population with many scheduling problems, but an especially effective art teacher. It would be useful to work with such an art teacher to solve the county-wide problems.
North Central	Poinciana Park Elementary	Emotionally Disabled	It was difficult for a regular art teacher to manage and serve these students because of the nature of the exceptionality.
South	Gulfstream Elementary	Autistic	The school had a large exceptional student education population. The regular art teacher was concerned about the difficulties that would be encountered in providing

| | | | meaningful art experiences for these students. |
| South | Merrick Elementary | Profoundly Mentally Retarded | It was difficult for a regular art teacher to manage and serve these students because of the nature of the exceptionality. |

5. Staff Development

To reinforce the information obtained from the school visitations, we extracted substantial information from a Staff Development Needs Assessment Survey which was distributed to all Dade County art teachers. Analysis showed that mainstreaming was the primary focus. The most essential topics were incorporated into the final content of the staff development program.

To assist in the development of the Art Education and Mainstreamed Exceptional Student Staff Development Module, planning meetings were held with two of Dade County's teacher-training support agencies: Florida Diagnostic Learning Resources System (FDLRS) and the Dade-Monroe Teacher Education Center (TEC). Both agencies helped identify potential workshop content, consultants, instructional materials, and supplementary financial resources.

We then planned a series of three staff development workshops for each administrative area. The general goals for the workshop series included:

- Developing an awareness of the creative process and its relationship with perception, cognition, and personality.
- Developing an awareness of the modifications required in art studio equipment to meet the special needs of disabled students.
- Developing an awareness of strategies and techniques for motivation and for art content.
- Exploring the relationship of visual arts education with the overall education of the mainstreamed exceptional student.

A countywide conference was planned as a culminating activity for the staff development module.

Workshop and conference sites were identified, and a year-long schedule was prepared.

Implementation

The art teachers were provided with preservice and inservice strategies and techniques for presenting art content to disabled students. Classroom management areas were addressed: student behavior, type of handicap and ways to deal with it, and coordination with exceptional student educators. On-site visitation experiences were drawn on to familiarize art teachers with the different ways in which other art teachers work with exceptional students. This preparation included an in-depth explanation of children's needs, the inner needs that govern the creative process, the application of professional skills in the field of art, and the possession of knowledge relative to normality and pathology in childhood.

Art experiences geared to disabled students were selected to strengthen specific areas of deficiency. Goals and objectives were developed to satisfy every type of disability. Questions that came up for consideration included: Can a teacher who is not familiar with the behavioral characteristics of emotionally distraught children solve their emotional problems and help them to grow? Can artistic creation alone alleviate an emotionally disturbed student's chaotic inner feelings manifested by acting out and other dangerous behavior? Will our art teachers be prepared to deal with emotionally disturbed students who manifest impaired ego functioning? Can the average art teacher provide adequately for profoundly disabled students, such as the retarded and the autistic? If disabled students were to receive a meaningful experience, answers to these questions had to be found.

Information was sought in the following ways:

1. Student Population

NOTE: Dade County was the fifth largest school system in the United States in the 1979–80 school year, with about 225,000 students. The approximate ethnic breakdown was 42 percent white, non-Hispanic; 30 percent Hispanic; 27 percent African American, non-Hispanic; and 1 percent other.

About 26,000 Dade County students were classified as exceptional (Dade County Public Schools, 1979). Thirteen exceptionalities were identified. The Pilot Program served the four different types of exceptionalities selected, with students ranging from 5 to 21 years of age. Each group of students attended special classes at the one school chosen in its own administrative area.

North Administrative Area—Physically Impaired Students

Biscayne Gardens Elementary School is located in the North Area of Dade County. There were 10 physically impaired children involved in the Pilot Program at this school. Students had muscular or neuromuscular disabilities that significantly limited their ability to move about, sit, or manipulate the materials required for learning; skeletal deformities or abnormalities that affected ambulation or posture and body use necessary in school work, because of temporary or chronic lack of strength, vitality, or alertness; or severe disabilities that substantially limited one or more of their major life activities.

North Central Administrative Area— Emotionally Disabled Students

Poinciana Park Elementary School is located in the North Central Area of Dade County. A class of seven emotionally disabled boys participated in the Pilot Program. These students often exhibited such consistent and persistent behavior signs as withdrawal, distractibility, hyperactivity ... and needed a special instructional program for all or part of the school day.

The emotionally disabled students typically showed an inability to learn, which could not be explained by intellectual, sensory, or general health factors; an inability to build or maintain satisfactory interpersonal relationships; inappropriate or immature types of behavior or feelings under normal conditions; a generally pervasive mood of unhappiness or depression; and a tendency to develop physical symptoms or fears associated with personal or school problems.

South Administrative Area—Autistic Students

Gulfstream Elementary School is located in the South Area of Dade County. A class of six autistic students participated in the Pilot Program. The students had severe disorders of communication, behavior, socialization, and academic skills. Their disability reflected some of the early developmental stages of childhood. They appeared largely to suffer from a pervasive impairment of cognitive and perceptual functioning, the consequences of which were manifested in limited ability to understand, communicate, learn, and participate in social relationships, as shown by extreme self-isolation and lack of eye contact; speech either lost or never acquired; sustained resistance to change in the environment and a striving to maintain or restore sameness; a background of developmental disability in which segments of normal, near-normal, or exceptional intellectual function might appear; a tendency toward head-banging, twirling, hand-shaking, rocking, or other self-stimulatory behavior; pre-occupation with particular objects, or certain characteristics of objects, without regard to their accepted function; and difficulty in developing symbolic thinking.

South Central Administrative Area— Profoundly Mentally Retarded Students

Merrick Elementary School is located in the South Central Area of Dade County. Five classes, each with seven profoundly mentally retarded students, participated in the Pilot Program. The students were severely impaired in intellectual and adaptive behavior, and their development reflected a significantly reduced rate of learning.

Collectively, the students exhibited all of the following characteristics, but individually they were as different from each other as are nondisabled people, and their range of competence was wide. Delayed intellectual growth was apparent, manifested by their immature reaction to their surroundings and by their impaired social response. Several children were nonverbal and extremely limited motorically; they required continual supervision and care. Many of them had additional handicaps, such as sensory deficiencies, cerebral palsy, epilepsy, or emotional disturbances, which served to intensify their severe developmental lags. However, some of the youngsters were able to develop minimal communication skills and to interact with the environment. A few were even able to communicate through primitive speech, gestures, and signs; to recognize familiar faces; to respond to simple commands; and to achieve some self-help skills.

2. Curriculum Goals and Student Art Experiences

a. Curriculum Goals

NOTE: The goals in this section are program goals and should not be confused with specific behavioral objectives for each child.

Goal 1: To provide opportunities for ten physically impaired students at Biscayne Gardens Elementary School to participate in weekly 60-minute art activities that would help them form positive self-concepts and become as physically independent as possible by developing learning in perception, manipulation, aesthetics, application, and artistic organization through experiences adapted to their special needs.

Goal 2: To provide opportunities for seven emotionally disabled students at Poinciana Park Elementary School to participate in weekly 60-minute art activities that would help them form positive self-concepts, control aggressive behavior, accept limits, tolerate frustration, work toward goals, and acquire self-confidence and self-respect related to learning and social interaction by developing learning in perception, manipulation, aesthetics, application, and artistic organization.

Goal 3: To provide opportunities for six autistic students at Gulfstream Elementary School to participate in weekly 60-minute art activities that were designed to foster the development of a positive self-concept, body image awareness, attentional skills, and language development.

Goal 4: To provide opportunities for 35 profoundly mentally retarded students at Merrick Elementary School to participate in weekly 60-minute art activities that could foster behavior management, sensorimotor skills, language development, self-help skills, and gross and fine motor skills.

b. Student Art Education Experiences

Activities to aid disabled students in meeting art objectives were developed in the format of Dade County's Art Education Curriculum, *CurriculArt* (1978). The guidelines were:

(1) The lessons were to take place once a week and to last for 60 minutes.

(2) The curriculum was to be correlated with the specific disability selected for each of the four schools and was to be coordinated with each student's Individualized Education Plan (IEP).

(3) Each group of students was to be served as a self-contained exceptional student education class.

(4) The art teacher or regular classroom teacher was to participate in the art experiences by offering assistance to the students in the form of encouragement and praise rather than through the performance of the work for the students. The teacher had an opportunity to observe the art therapist's approach to the students.

(5) The activities implemented with individual students were to be

influenced by the extent of each student's disabilities. Manual dexterity, coordination, self-concept, and physical independence were stressed with the Physically Impaired group. Controlling aggressive behavior, accepting limits, working toward goals, socialization skills, and self-concept were stressed with the Emotionally Disabled students. Kinesthetic manipulation, self-concept, language skills, and gross and fine motor skills were stressed with the Autistic group. Kinesthetic manipulation, hand-eye coordination, and motor skills were stressed with the Profoundly Mentally Retarded group.

3. Art Therapy Applications

    a. Art therapy procedures were followed once a week in each of the exceptionalities with selected individual students and groups.
    b. Emphasis was placed on the development of emotional maturity.
    c. Feedback was provided to teachers and parents.

4. Staff Development — Teacher Training Module

As has been noted, one of the main areas of emphasis in Dade County's Pilot Art Education Therapy Program was the implementation of inservice training for art teachers and other personnel interested in acquiring techniques and strategies for working with exceptional students.

Each staff development session was designed to lead to appropriate art instruction for exceptional students. Emphasis was placed on specific disabling conditions only when they made instructional differences. Teacher priorities were the foundation for the content of each staff development session, and mainstreaming needs were the primary focus. Ideas, methods, and resources for working with exceptional students in the mainstreamed classroom were explored in depth at each session. Heightening teacher sensitivity to the nature of various student conditions and structuring a learning-through-art environment which would be physically, psychologically, and emotionally supportive for the exceptional student were an integral part of each workshop presentation.

Responsibility for each workshop presentation rested on the Supervisor of Art Education and the Pilot Program Art Therapist. Tasks included the preparation of correspondence to inform art teachers and other interested personnel about the workshops scheduled for them in their area; about the planning, developing, and implementing of the instructional content; and about the seeking of consultants to provide some of the workshop presentations.

To determine the degree to which an objective had been achieved by the participants, questionnaire/reaction sheets were distributed at the end of each inservice session. After analysis of the information, the most pertinent material was incorporated into a workshop report.

The information that follows is a summary of the sessions that took place during the staff development program:

Workshop 1, "The Creative Process and the Handicapped Student," was designed to assist participants in developing an awareness of the creative process and its relation to child development. The key facts were that self-expression applies to all stages and levels of creative activity and that development of freedom of expression cannot be achieved without a study of what can be expected in modes of expression in the different age groups and on the different mental levels.

A slide commentary illustrated the stages of child growth and development in visual art products. Age-appropriate artwork, done by different children from ages 2 to 18, was shown. Characteristics of creative expression and psychological, emotional, and cognitive attributes were discussed for each developmental stage. Deviations from the norm were also discussed.

What was emphasized throughout the entire presentation was that disabled children experience the same stages of creative expression as their nondisabled peers; however, the rate of development may be slower for disabled children.

Workshop 2, "Art Materials and Tools," focused on appropriate adaptations of art studio equipment and art projects to meet the special needs of disabled youngsters.

Art project adjustments that had to be made in order to work with disabled students and types of studio equipment modifications were explored. A slide commentary illustrated some equipment adaptations and project adjustments.

Workshop 3, "Motivation and Art Content," gave workshop participants the opportunity to become familiar with the nature of some disabling conditions, types of activities appropriate for disabled youngsters, and strategies for motivation and behavior management. Hands-on experiences included activities designed to familiarize participants with the nature of different types of disabling conditions. Appropriate types of art projects to help remediate disabilities and strategies for dealing with students who are poorly motivated or who have behavioral problems were also discussed.

The staff development module not only included three workshops for each administrative area, but a countywide conference as a culminating activity of the staff development program. The conference was held on May 3, 1980. Titled "Visual Arts Education and the Mainstreamed Exceptional Student," the event was the second annual Learning Through the Arts Conference sponsored by the Dade County Public Schools together with the University of Miami School of Education and Allied Professions (Bush, 1980).

The countywide conference was the first major State of Florida conference to involve professionals in exploring the relationship between art education and art therapy in the overall education of exceptional students. Such crucial factors as funding of programs, training of teachers, delineation of responsibility, and specific teaching strategies were discussed. State and local school officials, university and public school educators, and art therapists participated.

PILOT PROGRAM CONCLUDING REMARKS

Art Education and Art Therapy gave the students a well-rounded program, adapted to their special needs, consisting of the application of art education principles and methodology in combination with art therapy techniques and strategies. The severely disabled children served in the program, who were originally identified as difficult for a regular art teacher to manage, had made excellent progress. An art therapist with a background both in art education and art therapy had provided effectively for these youngsters, demonstrating that one of the roles of an art therapist is that of a therapeutic art educator.

From the outset, the Pilot Program framework for evaluation was designed to describe and define the dominant characteristics of the program. No comparative or statistical information was gathered. Therefore, the information contained in this section does not convey the results of an experimental design. Rather, the results reflected are based on the experiences, observations, and judgments of the art therapist, the teachers, and the administrators, and are founded on documented evidence consisting of the many entries made for all of the components that comprised the Pilot Program. The results also reflect the fact that the

Pilot Program drew on the numerous experiences described in art therapy research prior to program implementation (Bush, 1980).

Observations and some general suggestions and teacher requests are included in the topics that have been consistently alluded to and that are summarized below.

1. Administrative Planning Meetings

Because the pilot program was a new program and a collaborative effort between the Division of Exceptional Student Education and the Division of Elementary and Secondary Education, and dependent on the school administrative areas for favorable outcomes, coordination and communication between the administrative offices were imperative. Support, input, approval, and emphasis on functions, roles, and tasks in each of the administrative settings were key factors affecting the success of the program.

2. Reporting Procedures

Since the pilot model was designed for potential replication and expansion for the following school year, it was essential that reporting procedures be maintained throughout the pilot stage. The preparation of written reports of meetings, staff development sessions, and student art experiences provided me (the Art Education Therapist) with a means of gauging progress and accountability for the program.

The development of reporting procedures was worthwhile, although maintaining current documentation presented some scheduling problems, as paper work often could not be completed on time. Although reporting was a lengthy procedure, once completed, the reports proved useful for tracking program management and for evaluating the accomplishments of the pilot program.

3. School Visitations

I visited sixteen schools/self-contained elementary art classes upon recommendation by the Executive Director of Exceptional Student Education, the Art Supervisor, and the Area Superintendents and their staffs. I found that:

a. Some art teachers lacked the techniques needed to present appropriate instructional content to disabled students.

b. Some art teachers had limited information on individual disabled students.

c. Some administrators had prepared inappropriate class schedules for art teachers. For example:

(1) One art class was scheduled after the other—each, in many instances, a different exceptionality requiring constant change of equipment, materials, and teacher approach.

(2) Many art teachers of self-contained classes had back-to-back schedules which left no time to move from one room to another.

(3) Limited time was allotted for the art lesson.

(4) Scheduling several groups from one exceptionality or from several exceptionalities together resulted in a class that was either too large or too diverse to teach effectively.

d. Some administrators had provided facilities that were too limited for the implementation of meaningful art programs.

e. Some administrators had not taken the needed competencies into consideration when hiring new art staff to fill vacancies at exceptional student education centers.

f. The Dade County Public School System formula of one art teacher to 730 students in allocating art teachers appeared unrealistic in schools with many self-contained classes of disabled students because 730 students in a regular school may mean 25 classes, while 730 students in an exceptional student center, where classes are small, may mean 35 to 40 classes.

g. In several cases, there was little communication between the art teacher and the exceptional student classroom teacher.

h. In some art classes of severely disabled children the art teacher had no assistance from the exceptional student teacher or from the aide who assisted in managing large numbers and difficult groups of youngsters.

Some art teachers expressed a desire for release time to observe other art teachers at work with exceptional youngsters. Most of the art teachers were convinced that they were not giving their self-contained exceptional students the maximum benefits of an art education because, as art teachers, they had little knowledge of the nature and limitations of the disabling conditions possessed by the students. Some art teachers felt that the autistic, profoundly mentally retarded, and emotionally disabled students in the self-contained classrooms presented the greatest difficulty.

Art therapists identified topics related to behavior management and the presentation of art content for mainstreamed students as a primary need in staff development sessions.

Of the sixteen classes visited, the art teachers in fourteen classes requested that their schools be selected to receive the services of art education therapy.

Of the two art teachers who did not want the services of art education therapy, one had a background in exceptional student education, and the other felt assured that she was providing an appropriate program for all of her students.

Overall, the goals of the visitations were achieved. I gained an awareness of specific needs, concerns, and approaches for art teachers, and of content areas for the staff development module. I also gathered information that would identify the potential schools/students that would receive the services of art education therapy.

4. Student Population Groups

In the course of the school year, administrators, art teachers, classroom teachers, and parents made comments about the population selected for the Art Education Therapy Program—the four groups of exceptional students in self-contained elementary art classes—the Physically Impaired, Emotionally Disabled, Autistic, and Profoundly Mentally Retarded.

   a. There was general agreement that the four exceptionalities selected for the pilot population were in need of special art education services.
   b. Several classroom teachers and several area and school administrators wanted *all disabled students* to be provided with appropriate art education therapy through the pilot program.
   c. There was general agreement that the students chosen for the physically impaired pilot class were developmentally age-appropriate, but that the relatively minor degree of disability experienced by a number of the students in that particular class would have suited them for the regular art classroom.
   d. It was felt that: art education for physically impaired students might not always necessitate specialized services by an art education therapist. With inservice training or instructional support, a

regular art teacher could often provide a meaningful program. The disabilities of most of the students chosen for the pilot program for the physically impaired were mild in nature. Their intellectual and language impairments were moderate, and their behavior self-disciplined. Although these students were in a self-contained art classroom, many of them could have been resourced into a regular art classroom. However, some of the students in the class were functioning within the trainable or educable mentally retarded range, and had learning limitations. For such students, as well as for the students who did have severe physical disability, specialized art education therapy services were appropriate.

e. It was agreed that the other three exceptionalities selected— Emotionally Disabled, Autistic, and Profoundly Mentally Retarded —represented severely disabled children. Because of the nature of their exceptionalities, these students appeared to be well-served in an art education therapy class with a specialized art curriculum and nonconventional teaching approaches and strategies adapted to meet their special needs. Also, although emotionally disabled students may have mild intellectual and language impairments, their behavior is disruptive in nature, and the autistic students have communication problems, behavior abnormalities, learning difficulties, and emotional dilemmas which are appropriately addressed in art education therapy. The profoundly mentally retarded students have severe intellectual and language impairments that require art education therapy.

It was concluded that the nature and degree of a disability should determine the extent to which specialized art education therapy services are administered in individual instances.

5. Curriculum Goals and Student Art Activities

The curriculum goals were designed in support of each student's prescriptive program under the Individualized Education Plan (IEP). The goals were suited to the students' exceptionalities, their educational programs, and their developmental levels.

All activities implemented with the students were either original lessons from CurriculArt or lessons adapted in the format of CurriculArt. Areas of art content and motivation were chosen for the developmental levels of the students. Overall, students were encouraged to develop competence and familiarity with materials, tools, and art processes by relating visual experiences to people, places, and things in the world. he creative expression of ideas, feelings, and moods was encouraged.

Physically Impaired

The CurriculArt lessons were quite effective with the physically impaired students. The curriculum was appropriately adapted to meet the special needs of some students who had such additional disabilities as low developmental levels, representative of mental retardation. When the curriculum was adapted, students with low developmental levels worked on the same content areas as other students, but were encouraged to complete as much work as possible. Allowing these students time to complete a project during following lessons was a key factor in the success of this program.

The selection of sequential art experience cards helped to establish the continuity of the lessons. Experiences based on a common factor, such as expression, were of critical importance in this program: e.g., many art experiences were based on imagination, and some utilized direct observation.

It was found that activities that involved manipulation and dexterity assisted the students in developing better coordination and physical independence. Several reports from the students, classroom teacher, aide, art teacher, and principal indicated that the students responded favorably to the activities and the supportive classroom environment.

Emotionally Disabled

Implementing some of the strategies of the regular classroom program was effective in the art program for the emotionally disabled students.

To deal with disruptive behavior, behavior modification techniques were employed through a structured token reinforcement and contingency contracting system. At times, behavior dependent on internal motivations was encouraged.

Various art experiences in the CurriculArt format included subject matter dealing with self-concept, family, school, and personal interest—how students related to themselves and their environment.

On several occasions students responded favorably to activities in which they silk-screened T-shirts. This was a lengthy project which helped encourage students to work toward a goal.

It was through art experiences that a symbolic freedom was possible for the emotionally disabled students—they were led to depict their feelings in art form and to talk about them. Allowing the students the opportunity to express their thoughts and feelings in a structured and supportive environment helped contribute to mastery over their feelings.

Periodic meetings with both the art teacher and the classroom teacher and reports confirmed that the students were receiving meaningful art experiences. A most important goal was accomplished, helping develop the students' behavior so that resourcing to other school classes would be possible.

It is my contention that many emotionally disabled children have unfulfilled needs. One emotionally disabled boy who was not enrolled in the art therapy component came to the art room one day during his breakfast period. He came purely of his own volition "just to use art materials." He wanted to know what he could do that was "bad" so that he, too, could have art therapy. It became apparent that the emotionally disabled students who were seen in art therapy were infused with enthusiasm which they shared with their peers.

Autistic

A structured and sequential art curriculum for autistic students complemented the teaching approach in their regular classroom. For example, the development of daily living skills was an important aspect of the classroom program, so art lessons were emphasized that related to body image and functioning, social awareness, and general orientation. Language and conceptual development were also a major aspect of the instructional program.

Overall, these students appeared to show great progress during the course of the school year. The development of eye contact, attentional skills, language, motor control, and familiarity with art materials, tools, and processes may be attributed, in part, to the art education therapy program.

Reports from the classroom teacher, assistant teacher, art teacher, and principal reflected considerable enthusiasm for the art therapy curriculum implemented with these students, as did the positive responses and educational advances made by the children.

Profoundly Mentally Retarded

The implementation of some of the strategies of the regular school program assisted in the effectiveness of the art activities conducted with the Profoundly Mentally Retarded students. For example, I worked with one student at a time, then had the aide or assistant teacher follow up by working with the same student. I integrated behavior management techniques, motor activities, language development, and self-help skills into each lesson.

The art program emphasized motor skills, and the use of tools, materials, and simple art processes. All art experiences were structured and repetitive, with minimal art concepts. Some entire lessons were spent on just painting to learn brush control and how paint covers the paper.

I found that the CurriculArt lessons were inappropriate for the Profoundly Mentally Retarded students. I therefore adapted certain concepts and strategies from the CurriculArt lessons and successfully implemented them by means of the special instructional approach.

The implementation of the specialized art curriculum for the profoundly retarded students afforded them an opportunity for discovery through structured guidance. Classroom teachers continually praised their accomplishment, efforts, and attention spans. Exploration with art media was a tool for communication and self-expression. Participation in the art activities provided a stimulus for personal growth. It clearly fostered the development of awareness through sensory stimuli.

6. Staff Development

The inservice program for art teachers and other personnel interested in acquiring techniques and strategies for teaching art to exceptional students addressed some major needs and concerns of the staff, as indicated by workshop reports and workshop reaction sheets.

Overall, the reports favored having personnel acquire knowledge and understanding of the value of art in the education of exceptional students, familiarity with goals and strategies of appropriate programming for mainstreamed students, familiarity with art areas and developmental stages of art expression, familiarity in identifying appropriate lessons that would promote involvement in the creative process, and the individualization of appropriate art activities.

Participants' completion of a workshop reaction sheet at the end of each inservice session measured workshop content, organization, consultant performance, and appropriateness, and provided a general assessment. The reaction sheets reflected satisfaction with the relevancy and conduct of the inservice program.

Teachers consistently raised significant questions related to providing on-site assistance and guidance for particular classes of mainstreamed youngsters during the 1979–80 inservice program. Personnel addressed the need for a demonstration model in which a consultant would be available to work directly with the art teachers and the groups of disabled students to provide experimental activities and feedback.

Since the staff development models had to be implemented in each of the administrative areas, workshop content had to be repeated four times, once for each administrative area, and a workshop report had to be repeated four times, once for each administrative area. I found it beneficial to learn from previous workshops when to alter or repeat strategies in each of the presentations; nevertheless, the repetition imposed a demanding schedule on me.

Most of the inservice sessions were presented on a Wednesday afternoon, which was the time designated in the Dade County Public Schools. Attendance was sparse at those sessions. Sessions were better attended on teacher workdays when teachers could arrange their time for the preparation of grade reports and various other teaching tasks, such as curriculum planning and development, as well as for staff development sessions.

The Learning Through the Arts Conference was the culminating event of the staff development module. It focused on the first major countywide effort to address the relationship between art education therapy and the education of the exceptional student.

PART TWO—THE POST PILOT PROGRAM

At the end of the 1979–80 school year, the Dade County Public Schools allocated funds for five art therapists for pilot program expansion during the 1980–81 school year. Four art therapists were employed, each of whom was to serve a select group of exceptional youngsters on the elementary level. Each therapist was assigned to one of Dade County's four administrative areas. I was the fifth art therapist, already on the staff. I monitored the elementary art therapy program and implemented a pilot program on the secondary level. A countywide staff development program was put in place.

Because art therapy was still a new program and a collaborative effort between several offices in the Dade County Public Schools, coordination and communication between school administrative offices remained imperative. Support, input, approval, and emphasis on functions, roles, and tasks in all of the four administrative areas were key factors in the success of the expanded program (Bush, 1981).

Since the pilot model was designed for replication, as well as expansion (Bush, 1980), it was essential that reporting procedures be maintained during the entire school year. The preparation of written reports of meetings, staff development sessions, and student art experiences provided the art therapists with a means of gauging progress and accountability for the program. Although a lengthy procedure, the reports proved useful for tracking program management and for evaluating the accomplishments of the program procedures. School visitations were also continued, which enabled many art teachers to receive hands-on teaching ideas and strategies. Staff development sessions were scheduled on a variety of topics that could help teachers better understand their students. Many of the sessions took place on teacher workdays, when no students were scheduled in school, or after school hours, making it easy for teachers to attend.

By 1985 there were eight art therapists in the Dade County Public Schools, working in a variety of school settings. Funding for the art therapists continued to come from the local school board budget. The program was shifted from its place under the administrative umbrella of the Art Education Office to the Division of Exceptional Student Education because an increasing number of students were being diagnosed as severely emotionally disturbed and because there were enriched funds to serve that population. It was a hard decision to make: stopping services for the other exceptional students who were receiving them—the autistic, the mentally retarded, and the physically impaired—and limiting the services to the emotionally disturbed, but at this point, administrators in exceptional student education had begun to ask for increased services for the severely emotionally disturbed students. Art therapy was needed more than ever before. It was both a novel and an inspiring situation—art therapy was in demand!

The severely emotionally disturbed students became the fastest growing population in the school system. Over 600 students were identified as severely emotionally disturbed out of a school population of approximately 230,000 (Dade County Public Schools, 1985). The service was viewed as a viable, effective, and important modality.

To serve the ever-growing number of students with severe emotional disturbance, the Dade County Public Schools began to contract with outside agencies. Several outside agencies worked with the system to provide psychological treatment and assessment services, including The Bertha Abess Children's Center and the Metro-Dade Department of Youth and Family Development. The art therapists were not part of the contracted personnel—they remained as locally funded school system personnel.

The format of art therapy in the Dade County Public Schools was adapted to meet the new focus: troubled, severely emotionally disturbed children, and the art therapists were each assigned to two school settings, to serve this population exclusively, offering their services at each site 2.5 days a week. With the psychologists, family therapists, social workers, and teachers who were provided, a school treatment team took shape. Programs for the severely emotionally disturbed were structured much like clinical day treatment programs traditionally found in a psychiatric agency or hospital-type setting even though many of them operated within a regular public school building or within an agency facility.

The art education component was eliminated from the schedule of the art therapists, providing them with more time to implement clinical art therapy objectives, the opportunity to see more individual students and small groups of students, and the increased time to do further assessment and diagnostic workups, as well as to meet with parents, teachers, and treatment team personnel to collaborate on student cases.

Several exceptional student education center programs hired their own art teachers with specialized training and interest in working with disabled students, and many school administrators sought professionals with specialized backgrounds to implement a meaningful art education program.

A number of people have inquired about what has happened to the shared philosophy of art education and art therapy that proved to be so successful during the pilot year. The philosophy remains as a viable and effective modality for serving youngsters with special needs. The Dade County Public Schools continues its effort to maintain art programming for disabled youngsters. There is an art teacher in every school in Dade County; that includes special education schools. There is also an art educator with exceptional education certification who coordinates staff development training programs with art for the disabled and with the special arts activities and projects, serving teachers and students in the entire school district. Personnel in the art therapy department are used to provide input, training, and consulting services as needs arise (Bush, 1990).

I coordinate the art therapy program as the department chairperson. This entails program management and consultation services for students and staff throughout the district. I also provide direct services, maintaining an ongoing caseload at one of the schools.

Today, the art therapy program has 20 full-time art therapists who are staff members of the Dade County Public Schools Division of Exceptional Student Education. Each therapist remains assigned to a site serving severely emotionally disturbed students. The title *Clinical Art Therapy Department* has been employed to emphasize the distinction between art therapy and the fields of *Art Education* and *Psychology* (Bush, 1993).

As the years have passed, program review has revealed that a number of the procedures implemented have been highly effective. We have been able to refine the procedures based on what has worked and what has not worked. Some of the success is attributable to the facts that:

- It became possible to determine which procedures had produced results during the one-year Pilot Art Therapy Program implemented in 1979.
- The number of art therapists available to meet the needs of emotionally disturbed students had increased after the pilot program was completed, and the results were reinforced in subsequent years.
- Progressive development of the pilot program has led to a program that has served as a model school system program in art therapy not only for the Dade County School District, but for other school districts, for the American Art Therapy Association (AATA), and for the National Art Education Association (NAEA).
- Staff development activities became an ongoing feature of instruction for art teachers, classroom teachers, psychologists, counselors, school administrators, and other interested personnel. The services of nationally known art therapists were often employed.
- Presentations were made at local, state, and national conferences and conventions, and the program, which became familiar to many people, received approval from a number of sources.
- Counseling departments from many schools that did not have an art therapist began to refer students for art therapy assessment.
- On-the-spot assistance was available to students referred by art teachers, classroom teachers, counselors, psychologists, and principals.

- Requests for help in hiring art therapists as contracted part-time personnel were received from school principals.
- Requests for information, consultation, and expanded services were received from school administrators.
- Requests for information and consultation were received from other individuals and school districts, both in the United States and abroad.
- Media attention increased locally and nationwide.

Much of my interest in art therapy has been realized through its development in the Dade County Public Schools. While an undergraduate student majoring in art psychology and education, I had seen a need for helping children in school settings. I had felt that art was a natural vehicle for communication. I had wondered: Was there a way to use art and intervention to help youngsters in crisis? Could art therapy serve as a preventive measure (Bush, 1976)?

After I encountered graduate students majoring in art therapy, I was able to study its applications with Don Jones at Harding Hospital, in Worthington, Ohio. Subsequently, I began graduate training with Dr. Myra Levick at Hahnemann Medical University, where my graduate thesis focused on art therapy in public schools. It was the first thesis at Hahnemann that studied art therapy in a public school setting.

I have learned subsequent to my early discoveries that art therapy belongs in the schools, both for regular and disabled students. From my success in creating situations in which art therapy can be utilized, I know that art therapy and public school education are a successful partnership. I know that, together, they can provide tools with which to engage students in self-expression and in emotional and cognitive growth. Although it is not my goal to cure children in schools, I believe that art therapy can treat their problems and can maximize their academic success. Even better, it can help them to help themselves. The task is great, but achievement will be greater still (Bush, 1994).

Chapter 5

HIRING CRITERIA FOR
SCHOOL ART THERAPISTS

The hiring of art therapists for work in school settings involves the considerable effort needed to locate individuals with the requisite credentials. The job market does not now have an oversupply of such professionals.

Training Requirements

One approach is a bachelor's degree with at least fifteen semester credits in studio art and twelve semester credits in psychology (including developmental and abnormal psychology), and a master's degree in art therapy.

Another approach is a master's degree in psychology or an allied field and twenty-one units of graduate art therapy studies (American Art Therapy Association, 1993).

NOTE: For those who wish to work in schools, coursework in school art therapy is suggested but not yet required, because school art therapy is not yet in general practice.

Proficiency

The American Art Therapy Association sets the standards for the awarding of credentials to professionally qualified art therapists. The Art Therapy Credentials Board, Inc. (ATCB), an independent organization, grants post-graduate registration (A.T.R.) after reviewing documentation of completion of graduate education and post-graduate supervised experience. The registered Art Therapist who successfully completes the written examination administered by the ATCB is qualified as Board Certified (A.T.R.–BC), a credential requiring maintenance through continuing education credits (American Art Therapy Association, 1995). For further information, you are referred to the documents published by the Art Therapy Credentials Board, "Adopted

Revised Standards and Procedures for Registration (Art Therapy Credentials Board, 1993).

The American Art Therapy Association believes that a registered and board certified art therapist meets qualifications equivalent to those certified for most related professions. However, many states require professionals who wish to work in a school to obtain teaching credentials. In all situations, applicants should have their A.T.R., or should be working on their A.T.R. In cases where art therapists teach art, aside from or in addition to therapy, state art teaching certification should be necessary. The American Art Therapy Association encourages each state to establish criteria for art therapists in the schools that align with current standards set forth by the association. State teacher certification boards and administrators should consider employing art therapists as related service providers with or without teaching credentials if they are equipped to provide a clinically oriented treatment program.

The Dade County Public Schools initially required art therapists with a master's degree in art therapy to have art education teaching credentials from the State of Florida as well. Art therapists who were hired without teaching credentials had to be certifiable; that is, they could work on the job with a temporary certificate and complete the art education requirements within a two-year period. Art education was viewed as a related field. The criteria were established because during the early years of the program, the art therapist's role was to teach art and do therapy. There were no other art therapists working in Florida schools then, and there was no educational certification or state of Florida license in art therapy. Five years after the program started, the work took on an exclusively therapeutic role—assessment and therapeutic treatment—which required only specialized clinical experiences.

In the early days, when art therapists were required to have art teaching credentials for the Dade County program, art therapists with a master's degree in art therapy and an undergraduate background in an area other than art education had to return to college, on their own time and at their own expense, to take six to thirty-six credits in art education courses. This was a time-consuming and costly investment, especially when these persons were already skilled and qualified to do the job they were hired for. Many individuals were not interested in returning to school to complete the additional coursework. The school system lost out on many professional applicants simply because the mechanism for hiring was geared to art education requirements, and state boards of education were generally not equipped to evaluate art therapy services or the art therapists who might apply them.

Today, the criteria for hiring art therapists in the Dade County Public Schools require that individuals have their registration credentials— A.T.R.–BC—or be in the process of acquiring credentials, and that they successfully complete the local agency application process and personal interview. Until Florida has a state art therapy license, teaching certification will be required; however, applicants may be certified in any area. This is usually based on the applicant's undergraduate preparation.

Professional Qualifications for School Art Therapists

School art therapists must be professionals with training in art therapy from an accredited graduate program in art therapy. Professionals should have a minimum of two years of experience with the child and adolescent populations. Experience in educational settings is desirable. Art therapists should maintain current credentials with the Art Therapy Credentials Board.

Salary Scale

Salary levels for art therapists in schools should be commensurate with those of other professionals in schools, including teachers and psychologists. For example, master's level and doctorate level art therapists should be paid what master's and doctorate level psychologists receive. Salaries should be scaled according to the number of prior full-time years of experience the art therapist has acquired in educational or clinical settings, including hospitals and special treatment programs.

Chapter 6

ROLES AND RESPONSIBILITIES OF
ART THERAPISTS IN SCHOOLS

The training and personal interests of individual art therapists predetermine the roles they feel prepared to perform. As the schools each have freedom to initiate their own programs, they are likely to hire people who will best serve their goals.

The roles that art therapists transact in a school situation, based on their training, expertise, and focus, and on the needs of a given school, may take the following forms:

- **Art Education Therapist.** Art therapists with a background in art education have the immediate ability to implement an art lesson, to identify pathological manifests in artwork, and to identify and treat potential problems. Severely disabled students, such as the autistic, the emotionally disturbed, and the profoundly mentally handicapped, must have an adapted art curriculum and nonconventional teaching approaches, and thus require art therapists who can teach art. Most of the art teachers are equipped to teach art to nondisabled students and cannot fulfill this role.
- **Clinical Art Therapist.** Clinical art therapists do not have to be certified art teachers because they do not teach. However, they have had studio art experiences in their training, and therefore have the requisite knowledge. The emphasis in this role is not on the art per se but on the use of art as psychotherapy—on the employing of therapeutic/diagnostic practices with children who have problems. Clinical art therapists can deal with regular education students and with exceptional education students. They can serve a regularly assigned caseload of students on a continuing basis.
- **Consultant.** Such art therapists perform the same duties as the clinical art therapists but on an individual referral basis.
- **Trainer.** These art therapists concentrate on staff development

for such school personnel as counselors, psychologists, and classroom teachers, to fill the gaps that exist in their knowledge with respect to child development. The inservice training is designed as a preventive measure. It enables school personnel, in their informal assessment of student artwork, to spot the cognitive and emotional problems of children at an early stage.

Schools that can employ art therapists equipped to carry out all of the roles would obviously be in a better position to offer a comprehensive program. However, the nonteaching art therapists are the ones who are most needed to meet the pressing problems of today's schools because the art therapists who do not spend their time teaching can spend the greater part of their time focused on the art therapy, leaving the art teachers to focus on the art education instruction. It should be noted here that art teachers are a normal complement of most schools. It should also be stressed that their services would take on greater value if they were better equipped to deal with special populations through training in college. That would assure each school a highly effective school team. The nonteaching art therapists on the school team would actually spend their time doing what they do best, identifying the emotional problems of the children by means of the children's artwork and then treating the children. The art teachers would carry out the art education duties currently required.

The application of art therapy can tie the work of the school team together. Other professionals on the school team cannot, professionally, link all the threads.

The job description of a school art therapist that follows can be adapted to individual school requirements:

1. Plans, organizes, and develops an art therapy program for the individually assessed special emotional needs of students from preschool through grade twelve.

2. Administers art therapy, provides documented assessments and followup interpretive conferences, and reports to interdisciplinary treatment teams.

3. Designs an individualized treatment plan for each student based upon information from the art therapy procedure and from the student's case history, reflecting the student's emotional and cognitive levels of functioning.

4. Carries out treatment plans by providing individual and small group art therapy services.
5. Assesses and documents the progress of students in art therapy.
6. Participates in meetings with interdisciplinary teams, collaborating with significant participants involved in case management.
7. Meets with parents, when possible.
8. Conducts inservice lectures, workshops, and presentations, and serves as a resource person to the staff regarding therapeutic intervention.
9. Performs administrative tasks, such as maintaining records, ordering materials and equipment, requisitioning supplies, and organizing the art therapy room.
10. Performs other assigned duties as required by the school program.

The current Dade County Public Schools Art Therapy Program engages in the application of personalized services to severely emotionally disturbed students. The clinical art therapists on the team work with the individual students and with groups of students. They collaborate with teachers and school psychologists, with other school support personnel, and with parents. They design and implement an individualized treatment plan for each student served. They utilize reporting procedures and write progress notes. The classroom instructional component and the art therapy component are considered to be equal partners in the process, contributing specific areas of professional expertise (Bush, 1995).

The overall aims of art therapy for a school system can be realized when:

A **Therapeutic Environment** has been established, and art therapists are conducting their art therapy at a physically and psychologically safe site. They have established a relationship with the students. They are adhering to health and safety regulations. They are providing structure and behavioral management. They are ensuring privacy and confidentiality.

Student Assessment has been performed and the art therapists have obtained information on family history and the events that precipitated contact with art therapy (medical, developmental, psychosocial, psychiatric). They have knowledge of the current level of functioning of the students and the students' mental status. They have evaluated the likelihood of any harm students might do to themselves or to others. They have discussed the assessment procedures with the students relative to art and to verbal and written tasks, and have identified student strengths and needs. They have reviewed the records of educators, social workers, psychiatrists and the school psychologists as needed. They have evaluated the appropriateness of art therapy as a treatment modality.

Treatment Planning has involved the formulation of art therapy treatment plans and goals, including treatment by other professionals, if necessary (physician, psychologist, psychiatrist), and discussions have been held with the other professionals.

Provision of Art Therapy Services has included the use of materials and equipment that encourage flexibility of self-expression. Art materials and processes have been adapted to the specific needs of the students. Students have been instructed in the use of art media. Inferences have been drawn regarding student affect, behavior, art products, comment, and verbal interaction during the art process. The use of the art process to explore feelings, thoughts, and perceptions, and to obtain feedback on increased self-perception, enhanced self-worth, and ego strength has helped to promote growth and healing. The art therapy pace has been based on the strengths and needs of the students. Student progress toward the therapeutic goals has been evaluated on a regular basis, and treatment plans have been modified as necessary. Consultation with professionals involved in specific cases has been regular, and students have been referred to other credentialed art therapists or mental health professionals, when appropriate. When termination has been required, the process has been facilitated to suit student needs and circumstances.

Documentation has been maintained on the initial assessment, the art therapy treatment plan, and student progress. Student artwork has been appropriately labeled with the student's name, the medium, content, and date of creation. Consent forms from the family or guardian for the release of student artwork and release forms submitted by applicants for the use of the artwork have been kept on file. Written reports have been prepared, as needed, for the courts, the youth and family service agencies, and the professionals involved in student treatment.

Professionalism and Ethics have been an integral part of all action. Art therapy services have been provided in accordance with the AATA Code of Ethics for Art Therapists (AATA, 1994), the AATA General Standards of Practice Document (AATA, 1994), and the policies and procedures of the school district. Originals and copies of student images have been retained in a secure and confidential manner. Students have been engaged in self-appraisal on an ongoing basis. Contact has been maintained with a network of professionals, and the art therapy services have been in compliance with federal, state, and local regulations regarding business practices and the provision of mental health services. State and local laws have been complied with regarding reports of physical or sexual abuse and neglect. Students and families have been informed about community activities available to them in the areas of art, education, and leisure pursuits. Inservice training has been provided for the art therapists and other mental health professionals, and lay persons have been educated on the need for the practice of art therapy.

When art therapy services are broadly implemented and a school district has the benefit of a department chairperson to coordinate services, as in Dade County, the department chairperson is responsible for the planning, organizing, and monitoring of the art therapy services.

The duties of the Art Therapy Department Chairperson in the Dade County Public Schools are outlined as follows:

- Develops plans for the provision of districtwide art therapy services.
- Monitors the implementation of the art therapy services.
- Analyzes human, fiscal, and material needs for implementation of the art therapy program.
- Develops and monitors long- and short-term program goals to facilitate the provision and the improvement of the art therapy support services.
- Collects data for monitoring the effectiveness of art therapy.
- Provides technical support for art therapists.
- Conducts program observations at the school level.
- Prepares and submits records and reports to school-based and other exceptional student administrators, as required.
- Provides direct technical assistance to principals who have art therapy programs.
- Develops and disseminates documents pertaining to art therapy program procedures.
- Recruits potential art therapy personnel.
- Provides support and assistance to District Exceptional Student administrators who are responsible for art therapy personnel evaluations and audits.
- Develops budget proposals and monitors expenditures.

- Develops, monitors, and implements staff development for art therapists and other interested school personnel.
- Conducts regular departmental meetings for the purpose of sharing information, discussing problems that may arise, and assisting personnel in updating art therapy techniques and strategies.
- Keeps staff members up to date on new or changed procedures that affect the completion of their duties, the maintenance of their skills, and the updating of their knowledge.
- Maintains a link between the district and the regional offices in the implementation of the art therapy services.
- Plans, organizes, and develops procedures designed to meet the individually assessed special needs of the exceptional education students in the program.

I have continued to provide direct service to selected students, in addition to my supervisory functions.

Art therapists are self-directed with respect to the functions they carry out at individual job sites. Theoretically, they can be expected to adjust their focus to suit the needs of any given institution. Through the kinds of teamwork I have described, they can become an integral part of a school system.

Chapter 7

IDENTIFICATION, ASSESSMENT, AND SCHEDULING OF STUDENTS

Public Law 94-142, The Education for All Handicapped Children Act (1975), and the Individuals with Disabilities Education Act, Public Law 101-476 (1990), refer to children who are learning disabled, emotionally disturbed, hearing impaired, speech or language impaired, visually impaired, seriously emotionally disturbed, mentally retarded, and orthopedically impaired, and to children who are autistic, or who suffer from traumatic brain injury or another incapacitating impairment. The pressing needs of these youngsters call for particularized educational applications. Under the law, individuals recognized as disabled qualify for special education and related services.

Based on national lobbying efforts, the Senate Report on the Code of Regulations for Public Law 94-142 clearly defined art therapy as a related service that could assist a disabled child to benefit from education (Section 121a.305).

There are likewise a number of children who have not been identified as disabled but who have difficulty at school owing to social or emotional problems stemming from a crisis at home, such as the death of a significant person, parental separation or divorce, or physical abuse. I believe that students who have not been identified as disabled stand to profit from art therapy treatment in equal measure.

Art therapy is equipped to offer a therapeutic, diagnostic/prescriptive approach to students who have been identified as disabled and to students who may be identified as disabled.

IDENTIFICATION

Student Selection for Art Therapy

Procedures for referring and placing students in art therapy accord with the guidelines established by each school for all of its youngsters receiving special services. However, art therapy should not necessarily be prescribed based on the availability of the service, but on need.

It may not be possible for the art therapist to see every student who needs treatment, but, so long as school personnel are familiar with art therapy, and can recognize the kind of student who would benefit most from the therapy experience, there should be no problem.

The following list of characteristics, or indicators, can help to determine the suitability of a student for art therapy. The list merely highlights certain features that are often recognizable in art therapy candidates.

- Behavior problems are manifested within the school milieu: for example, excessive absences, adjustment difficulties, peer pressure, poor peer interaction, difficulty with authority figures.
- Other behavioral manifestations exist, such as irritability; unhappiness; depression; anger; withdrawal; foreign language barriers; excessive verbal or nonverbal communication; disruptive, destructive, and aggressive behavior; insecurity; lack of self-confidence; inappropriate or no affect; poor self-image; excessive use of fantasy.
- Serious emotional or traumatic experience is associated with the nonschool environment: crisis in the home, death of a significant person, parental separation or divorce, physical or mental ailment, physical or psychological abuse.
- The student has difficulty expressing thoughts and feelings verbally, and appears to express thoughts and feelings more easily through art.
- The student is generally withdrawn and does not seem to be a good candidate for verbal therapy.
- The student shows a desire and willingness to participate in art therapy.
- Observations of the artwork by the art therapist show danger signs in the student's artwork.

Individualized Education Plan (IEP)

The Individualized Education Plan (IEP) is an annual plan of instructional and support services that will assist the student in reaching educational goals. If art therapy is applied to a youngster receiving exceptional education services, documentation of the art therapy experience as a related service must be indicated on the Individualized Education Plan. The art therapist should: Indicate that art therapy is a related service, the date the service will begin, and the length of time the service will take. Document the student's current level of functioning. Give an annual art therapy goal and short-term objective. Document the length of individual and/or group sessions. Provide schedules, procedures, and objective criteria for annual evaluation, and a description of the art therapist service provider (Morreau and Anderson, 1984). There is an additional section, recently added by IDEA (The Individuals with Disabilities Education Act), which requires a transition plan for students 14 years of age and older (P.L. 101-476, 1990).

If an IEP has been prepared, a meeting to review the student's progress is planned annually. At that time, the IEP is reviewed by the student's parents or guardians and by school administrators and teachers, and, if necessary, updated. The art therapist should be present at this meeting in order to discuss the student's progress and need for termination or continued treatment.

If art therapy is provided to a youngster not served in the exceptional student program, it is suggested that a similar format of planning and review of services be followed.

Procedures for completing IEP forms and the forms themselves vary from school district to school district. It will be up to the art therapist to implement procedures with a structure the school program offers. An abridged version of the Regulations and Procedures for the IEP is given in Appendix A.

ASSESSMENT

The school art therapist is advised to implement a diagnostic art therapy assessment that ascertains the cognitive and emotional development of the youngster. An assessment can help to determine the appropriateness of the student placement in art therapy as well as provide base line data on the student, and serve to establish goals and objectives for treatment. The assessment may be implemented prior to placement in a special program, in conjunction with the psychological testing process, or it may be used after the youngster has been placed in a special program to provide further information about the youngster. Schools are advised to implement the procedures that would be most beneficial to their programming needs.

The Dade County Public Schools Art Therapy Program took part in the development of the Levick Emotional and Cognitive Art Therapy

Assessment (LECATA), which was developed in the spring of 1989. Members of the program collaborated with Myra Levick, a nationally known expert in the field, to develop the procedure (Levick et al., 1989).

The LECATA is a comprehensive six-task drawing assessment that focuses on both the emotional and cognitive development of an individual. It provides the significant indicators in one tool. It is designed to reveal unique, important, and valuable information to the school treatment team that is otherwise not available. This information gives the team an understanding of the developmental level a child is functioning at, or that the child may regress to, and the potential of the child to achieve. A sample parental consent form to conduct an art therapy assessment is shown in Appendix B, and a sample assessment report is shown in Appendix C.

Goals and Objectives

The goals and objectives are the treatment plans for the students. A student's goal and objectives, extracted from the assessment, provide a listing of the emotional and cognitive expectations planned in art therapy for that school year. The goal and objectives should be written on a student's IEP.

A sample copy of a goal and objectives report may be found in Appendix D, and sample guidelines for developing goals and short-term objectives may be found in Appendix E.

Progress Report—Post Year Assessment

A progress report provides data on the results of the art therapy received during the school year. One of the tasks from the initial assessment is administered, and the score and results are reported in terms of the student's growth and development during the school year. The report is completed annually and filed by May 30 of each school year or when a student terminates art therapy, if that is earlier than May 30.

A sample copy of the progress report appears in Appendix F.

Transfer of Information on Assessment Results

Upon completion of all reports, art therapists should verbally share the results with appropriate program staff, including the student's classroom teacher and other clinicians assigned to the case. A forum for sharing may include a case conference meeting or meetings, arranged with individual personnel. A sample copy of a Case Conference report form may be found in Appendix G.

If clerical support is available, all documentation should be typed.

Student artwork (original or photocopy) must be attached to the appropriate report and labeled with the student's name and date. Pertinent directives should be included. It is not necessary to include artwork with the student's Goal and Objectives Report or in the IEP.

Reports are filed as follows: A copy of the report with the original artwork is filed in the art therapist's files; one copy of the report with photocopied artwork is filed in the student's educational cumulative record; and one copy of the report with photocopied artwork is filed in the program clinical case file if the case is in a special clinical program.

If a student transfers to another school, the art therapist should ensure that the appropriate art therapy reports follow the student to the new school. Just as psychological reports are transferred with a student's records, art therapy reports, which provide documentation on the student's condition, should be transferred.

SCHEDULING

In Dade County, one art therapist is assigned to a school site to provide services for a caseload of approximately 20–25 students a week. The art therapist prepares the schedule with the input of members of the clinical and teaching staff.

The time suggested for sessions is 60 minutes for assessment evaluations, 30 to 45 minutes for each individual session, and 45 to 60 minutes for each group session.

The art therapy schedule of services will vary depending on available facilities—whether there is a separate room fully equipped, or there is no designated art therapy room; scheduling factors—the student's individualized schedule, the teacher(s) schedule(s), the art therapist's schedule, the schedules of other service providers; and the assessed needs of individual students—their levels of cognitive functioning, emotional functioning, physical maturity, social behavior, and academic functioning.

A sample copy of a schedule appears in Appendix H.

SESSION TREATMENT PLAN

Session planning is an essential part of the art therapy process. Procedural objectives for a session should be an extension of the goal and objectives of the IEP, extracted from the art therapy assessment. Session plans provide a long-term goal, a short-term objective, materials, evaluation of the session, and followup strategies.

A sample copy of a session treatment plan appears in Appendix I.

Chapter 8

TREATMENT OUTCOMES

Drawings open a door to hidden feelings, revealing issues to the art therapist that are not easily expressed in speech. Most people respond well to the use of drawing in art therapy. Creative individuals, who already use art for self-expression, respond especially well to the use of drawing in art therapy. Nonverbal, withdrawn, resistant youngsters find it easy to express their thoughts and feelings through art products because art gives them a vehicle for communication that does not force them to talk. Rageful youngsters who may be afraid of being overwhelmed by their anger find a safe outlet in drawing, which causes the threat of becoming destructive to recede. Students of many types can actually resolve conflicts through the art therapy medium that might otherwise never be addressed. Making art, and talking about it, may be the best means a variety of students have of expressing themselves; in some cases, the only means.

As children grow, they develop verbal fencing skills that enable some of them to avoid facing their real problems. The use of art materials can force such children to lower the walls that have enclosed them and that have prevented them from expressing their needs to others. They can drop the defensive postures that have kept them from relating to others on a personal level; they can begin to develop relationships, and even, later on, a sense of intimacy with others. Developing intimacy may be a far-reaching goal; it is the loss of intimacy and the inability to attain it after a damaging early experience that have precipitated these children into the kinds of problems from which they have been referred for treatment. If the first intimacy that they can achieve is with themselves through the art that they make, then we have started them on the path to achievement in their lives.

The following three cases illustrate the promising results the art therapy treatment programs have produced in public school classrooms.

NOTE: The names of individuals have been changed to insure privacy.

THE CASE OF CARLOS

By Jennifer Lombroia

Carlos is a seventh grade student at a Miami, Florida, public school serving approximately 200 severely emotionally disturbed and emotionally disabled middle school students. The school pursues an interdisciplinary program offering a myriad of services. I am on the staff of its clinical department. I am a clinical art therapist. Also on this staff are a psychiatrist who treats children and adolescents, school psychologists, social workers, and counselors.

Carlos is a handsome, 13½-year-old, solidly built, Hispanic male with a fair complexion and dark, curly hair. He is outgoing and personable, yet quick tempered. He is popular among his peers and greatly admired for his artistic talent. He has been hospitalized twice since the age of 10 for depression, aggressive behavior, and suicidal ideation. Following his first hospital stay, he was placed in a program for severely emotionally disturbed students, where he completed the fourth grade.

Carlos came to the United States from Puerto Rico with his mother and older stepbrother, when he was 3½ years old, to flee a father who was a violent and abusive alcoholic. His mother stated that her husband had physically abused her and the children, and that she had required hospitalization for a seizure disorder caused by blows to her head. Three months after Carlos, his mother, and stepbrother came to the United States, Carlos's father died of a heart attack.

The mother's pregnancy with Carlos had been difficult because of the emotional and physical abuse inflicted by her husband. She had been diagnosed with carcinoma of the cervix, and an abortion had been recommended. In spite of this, Carlos was born, but with complications. Shortly after his birth, his mother had been hospitalized for a kidney operation. She had remained in the hospital for a month. Upon returning home, she had, reportedly, suffered from a psychotic episode and had been treated unsuccessfully with antipsychotic medication. She stated that for approximately one year she had had difficulty responding to the needs of Carlos, and had little awareness of his developmental milestones during that period. She has experienced two or three psychotic episodes since the first one, which Carlos has witnessed.

Carlos currently lives with his mother, who has recently separated from his stepfather. His stepbrother, with whom he has had a close relationship, has married and left home. Contact with him has since been minimal, which has been a disappointment to Carlos. His relationship with his stepfather has been strained, and Carlos has expressed relief that the stepfather has moved out of the house.

Prior to placement in this school, Carlos had been recommended for art therapy by the art therapist at his former school, who had found it to be an effective intervention for him. According to her art therapy assessment report, Carlos had demonstrated the ability to use cognitive skills close to his chronological age, but his combined average score at that time reflected a developmental level of 6.4 years of age.

Some of the themes mentioned in the original assessment, repeated in Carlos's artwork over the past year and a half, have related to feelings of loss, sadness, and unresolved grief. In one of the tasks, "A Place of Importance," Carlos drew a "cemetery" in pencil, and stated, "A sad place, that is why I don't want to tell you . . . in Puerto Rico in Tohando in San Juan he (father) died when I was three years old. I can't express sadness so that's when I get mad and throw things." The drawing (Figure 1) depicts an isolated figure placing a flower on a grave; the figure is devoid of hands, feet, and facial features. Depression and unresolved grief are evident in this drawing.

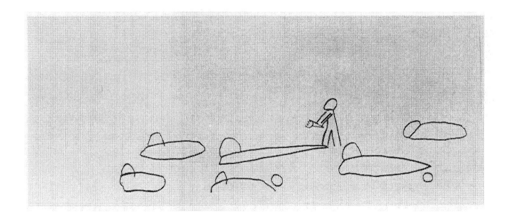

Figure 1. Grieving Figure (Carlos).

Carlos had learned early on in therapy how to use his artistic talent and insight to understand and communicate what he was experiencing emotionally. These skills became valuable tools that were effective in helping him to strengthen his coping skills while learning to express sadness and to accept the losses in his life, and, in the process, to develop a stronger self-concept. An ongoing theme in therapy has been the intense anger and sadness he has experienced as a result of the many losses in his life, and the difficulty he has in controlling his feelings and expressing them appropriately. During one of the first sessions we had, he was very open about why he had been hospitalized and placed in an SED (Severely Emotionally Disturbed) program. He realized how powerful an emotion anger could be and the importance of learning how to express and channel it in ways that would benefit him rather than hurt him. Art became a valuable outlet for him. His emerging identity as an artist was a way for him to connect and relate to me. He was self-motivated and eager to participate in art therapy, and responded well to a nondirective approach. His proclamation, "My art is me!" was in many ways a metaphor for the development of his personality.

Carlos's artwork focused on familiar feelings of anger and sadness, both past and present. This was a time when the marriage of his mother and stepfather was rife with conflict, and he was thinking more and more about returning to his family in Puerto Rico, "where people don't hate each other." He created a mask (Figure 2) as a symbol of his anger and hurt, and after completing it, stated "This was when I was still mad but starting to control my anger." He was beginning to recognize that his aggressive outbursts covered over his sadness, which was more difficult for him to express. Shortly after completing the mask, he created another one (Figure 3) which revealed a more fragile and delicate side of himself. It portrayed a sad and crying person and, according to Carlos, symbolized the "sadness in my life."

Carlos was beginning to talk more about his past and about his relationship with his family in Puerto Rico and New York. He talked about the isolation he felt owing to the absence of extended family in Miami. His stepbrother's recent marriage and move from home had been another source of loss in his life, and he continued to express his desire to be with aunts, uncles, and cousins either in Puerto Rico or in New York.

It was during this time in therapy that he discovered both a talent for three-dimensional media and the inherently expressive quality of clay. He began a series of clay figures which symbolized and affirmed a gradual yet dramatic emergence of a stronger sense of self. While working on his first sculpture, "Man of Prayers" (Figure 4), he began to talk about when he was younger and had an uncontrollable temper. He said

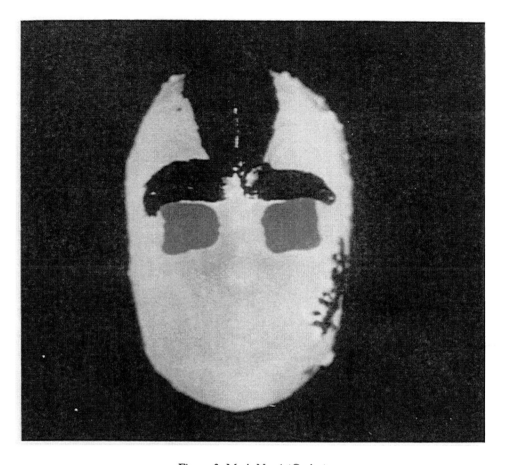

Figure 2. Mask No. 1 (Carlos).

he used to wish he were an animal because he "acted like one," and he wished he could go back and change his past. The sculpture expressed great sadness and revealed a vulnerability which, he stated, few people recognized as a part of him. It reflected fragility, yet revealed an inner strength and control that were beginning to develop. He was having fewer fights with peers and was becoming more involved in school activities. Another positive factor was his participation in an art class with a male teacher, whom he admired, and with whom he was beginning to identify.

Shortly after he completed the "Man of Prayers," Carlos's grandmother in Puerto Rico passed away. It had been only two years since his grandfather had died, and he had had a close relationship with both of them. He attended the funeral, and upon his return was quite open

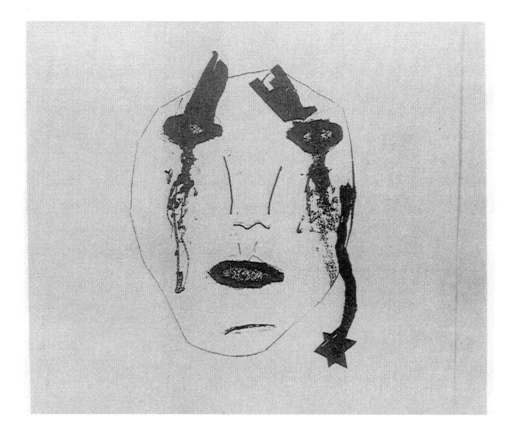

Figure 3. Mask No. 2 (Carlos).

regarding the experience. What seemed to affect him more than his grandmother's death was his mother's irrational and hysterical behavior during the funeral, and her threat to jump into her mother's grave. Carlos began to talk more about his mother who, in his mind, was the weakest and most fragile of her brothers and sisters. He began to recognize and accept her limitations, and seemed better able to express sadness and resolve about the experience.

Carlos continued to work with clay and created another figure (Figure 5) kneeling and kissing the ground. He entitled it "Sad—that's all I have to say," but later referred to it as a symbol of his "weak and tortured self." He had been learning to cope with the ongoing conflicts between his mother and stepfather, which resulted in improved academic and behavioral performance. He began another sculpture (Figure 6) that he

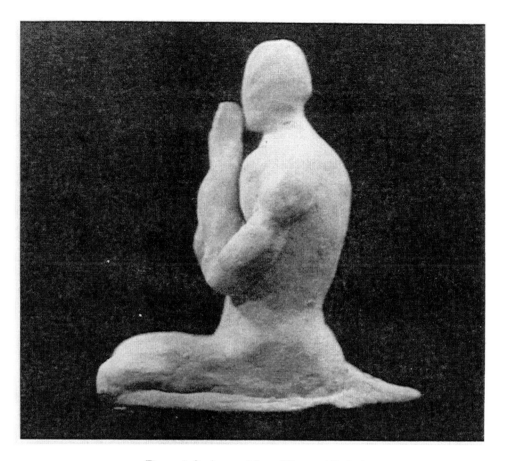

Figure 4. Sculpture–Man of Prayers (Carlos).

described as "strong." He was learning to talk more about the traumatic events in his life and was beginning to put them behind him. His identity as an artist was growing, and his skill in controlling and constructively channeling his anger was increasing. Upon completion of this sculpture, he described it as himself, "When I'm strong and healthy . . . and no one can hurt me anymore."

Carlos's progress was dramatic. Art therapy, I believe, was a haven through which he could learn to trust and develop himself in new ways. He became more emotionally stable and, as a result, was able to succeed in the classroom environment. Like the clay sculptures he created, he learned to mold, shape, and create a strong identity. Art therapy gave him an opportunity to express and gain more control over his emotions and, in the process, his life.

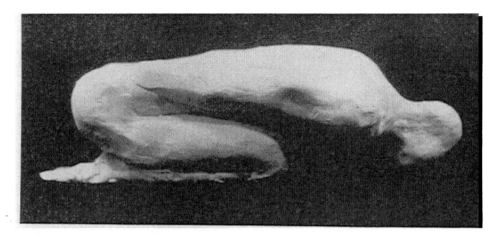

Figure 5. Sculpture–Figure Kneeling (Carlos).

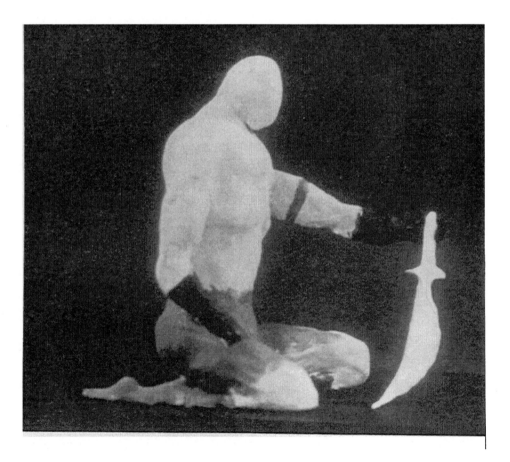

Figure 6. Sculpture–Strong (Carlos).

THE CASE OF JAKE

By Sarah P. Hite

In Hampton Roads, Virginia, a private day school meets the needs of special education students who have exhausted the resources of their public school system. Most of the students are classified as Seriously Emotionally Disturbed. The day school offers a range of services and interventions to facilitate the successful transition of students to a less restrictive academic environment in the public school setting. Services include a 7:2 student:teacher ratio; a thematic, sequential curriculum; family support groups; vocational assessment and preparation; speech and language services; art therapy; and individual, group, and family counseling.

The art therapist, who works within the counseling department, is called an Expressive Arts Counselor. Her role includes art therapy assessment, individual and group expressive arts counseling (art therapy), IEP (Individualized Education Plan) development, home visits and in-home family intervention, and liaison work with community agency and referring school system personnel. The art therapist and the other clinical counselors at the day school all function as primary therapists.

Jake, a fifteen-year-old Caucasian male, was referred to this day school because of problem behaviors that prevented even marginal success at public school. He fought with peers, threatened school authorities, was disruptive and noncompliant in his self-contained classroom, and took dangerous risks on the school bus. He had had similar problems dating back to the first grade, at which time he was determined to be eligible for special education services as an emotionally disturbed (SED) student.

Jake's difficulties in academic settings are a function of emotional disturbance rather than cognitive deficits or learning disabilities. He is the middle child in a blended family. At present, he resides with his mother and stepfather. An older half-sister, from his mother's first marriage, lives away from home, and a younger brother, Matt, is in residential treatment. Jake and Matt's father abused all three children sexually when Jake was 5 to 7 years old. His father's whereabouts are unknown, and there has been no contact for years. After the abuse was discovered, and outpatient intervention failed, Jake was hospitalized for six weeks.

His psychiatric diagnosis was Dysthymic, with Mixed Specific Developmental Disorder on Axis II. After the hospitalization, the siblings were separated. Jake and Matt were placed together in a foster home several hundred miles away; the sister was placed in residential treatment. Jake's understanding is that the placements were initiated by his mother, who "could not handle" the children, and who "needed time to get her life together" with her third husband. The foster placement lasted about two years, after which all three children lived together with their mother and stepfather until the time of Jake's referral to day school. Jake's extreme hyperactivity was addressed through medication prescribed by the family doctor, but inconsistently administered by his mother. Jake attributed his rate of academic success to medication, rather than to his ability.

At the day school, Jake was assigned to the art therapist for individual work. The art therapy assessment revealed that Jake fluctuated between latency and adolescent levels of adjustment—cognitively, socially, and emotionally. An impaired sense of self, with feelings of hopelessness, a sense of powerlessness, and a lack of internal locus of control, was expressed verbally and manifested in his drawings. Human figure drawings included crosshatching in the pelvic area (Figure 7), suggesting anxiety associated with sexuality. Depression was noted in Jake's verbalizations and through the lack of color, movement, and detail in his drawings. Verbalized problems with anger management were not reflected in the assessment drawings. However, impulsivity was manifested through task approach as well as through lack of necks in the drawings, and heads attached directly to bodies, suggesting an inability to separate thought from action. He appeared to behave impulsively in response to internal tensions rather than as the result of thinking about or reflecting upon inner experience. What appeared most consistently in the assessment drawings was Jake's coping style, which included wholesale avoidance of his inner world through the use of denial and isolation of affect.

Individual art therapy, through which Jake could objectify his conflicts and problem areas, thus making them available for consideration and processing during the sessions, seemed the ideal therapeutic approach with this impulsive, avoidant student. However, his history of abuse, coupled with abrupt and chaotic separations and losses, suggested significant problems with trust. A therapeutic alliance, upon which successful treatment progress hinged, would be difficult to achieve with Jake. An

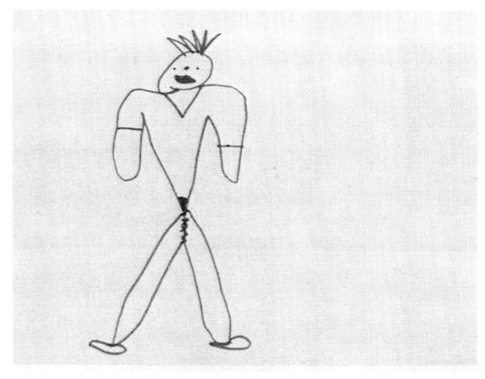

Figure 7. Self (Jake).

IEP, which included the following objectives, was prepared: (1) Develop a productive counseling alliance, based upon trust, which involves an understanding of the benefits and limitations of the counseling process; an appreciation of expressive arts counseling as a tool for emotional, social, and cognitive growth; and an acknowledgment that artworks produced in sessions are self-projections. (2) Increase self-knowledge through the exploration of self-image, values, and experiences; the examination of personal history impact on present functioning and self-concept; and the expansion of a repertoire of appropriate expressions of affect. (3) Increase responsibility for behaviors—to show increased understanding of the effect of feelings upon behaviors; decreased impulsivity; and consolidation of the internal locus of control. It was hoped that attainment of the objectives would lead to a more positive self-concept and increased ability to make logical success-oriented choices.

Jake's schedule included one sixty-minute session a week. Throughout the school year, 37 regularly scheduled sessions and 6 crisis sessions were held. It is noteworthy that although Jake was disruptive in school, that he had difficulty concentrating on his academic subjects, and that he wandered in and out of the classroom, he was consistently focused in his sessions. Artwork he produced in the sessions eloquently illustrated the issues and themes that emerged in the treatment process.

The prevalent theme of the first 12 to 15 sessions was that of trust versus mistrust regarding the therapeutic relationship, manifested in the house Jake constructed using craft sticks, tempera, sequins, glitter, and pipe cleaners (Figure 8). During the hours devoted to this project, Jake explored the parameters of the counseling situation, expressing concern about confidentiality, sharing information about past failed treatment efforts, complaining about the unequal nature of the student-counselor relationship, questioning the validity of the art therapy process, and verbalizing his inability to trust anyone at all. Midway through construction, he noticed with surprise that his house had no doors or windows, but he made no effort to add them. Finally, he added sequins to the roof, which he said were "solar catchers to collect warmth from the environment," and a pipe cleaner as an "antenna to receive signals from the outside." Through his house, Jake had expressed his apprehensions and his fears, as well as his ambivalence about engaging in a treatment alliance.

A second significant theme was that of Jake's powerful and disturbing anger and its relation to self-mutilation and other aggressive and impulsive behaviors. One aspect of this theme was the issue of internal versus external locus of control, including the impact of untempered impulses upon behavior. This theme was developed both in regular weekly sessions and in unplanned crisis-oriented sessions. Jake's wood sculpture (Figure 9) proved to be a vehicle for the cathartic expression of his rage through forceful hammering and pounding. Making this object provided Jake with an opportunity to understand the impact of decisions upon the final product, through technique and construction, and served as a metaphor for creating order out of chaos.

The creation and processing of the molded plaster sculpture (Figure 10) proved pivotal in terms of Jake's understanding of the treatment process. The nature of the task dictated a collaborative effort, and through it, Jake learned that working together yielded a product impossible to achieve alone. The casting was conceived and executed horizontally, i.e., Jake had his hand extended from his waist, palm up. This supplicant-like position inspired conversation in which Jake weighed the risks and

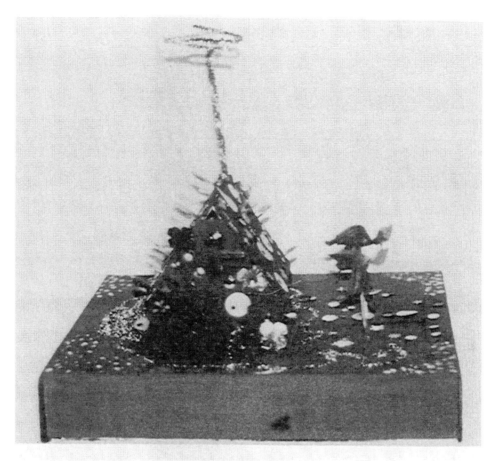

Figure 8. House (Jake).

benefits associated with asking for help. Painting and finishing the project required placing the casting upright. In that position, it inspired an association of power, rage, and aggression. At this point, Jake was cutting his forearm with a razor blade; the cuts are represented on the sculpture with sequins. Making this formed plaster sculpture afforded Jake an opportunity to understand the function of his self-mutilation: he was displacing the rage felt toward others onto himself. Throughout the rest of the academic year, Jake continued to gain and internalize insights about the anger within him. The result was greater impulse control, a decrease in problem behaviors, and increased self-esteem.

In the spring of the academic year, the art therapist prepared reports aimed at justifying tuition for a second year's placement at the day school, disseminating the reports to the appropriate public school and

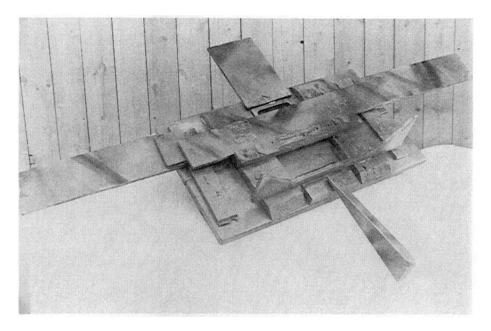

Figure 9. Wood Sculpture (Jake).

community agency personnel, and then advocating continued funding at a series of meetings. After funding was approved, Jake and the art therapist worked together to review the year's work, to summarize gains, and to develop plans for the following year.

The Inside-Outside Box (Figure 11), pictured with the lid resting on the bottom, is the last project Jake completed before summer break; it dictated a focus for future work. On the outside of the box lid, Jake represented, with glitter, feathers, and gems, the charming, engaging social self he often displayed to others. The sandpaper covering the sides symbolized his reluctance to allow others entrance into his inner world. The inside of the box, representing his inner self, was lined with feathers and plastic pop paper "for protection of breakable things." A tiny inner box, constructed of sandpaper and sealed shut with glue, contained the words "Help me." Bits of colored paper symbolized the gains made during this year of intensive art therapy treatment. While previous artworks had been created somewhat spontaneously, then processed and related to current struggles, this carefully thought-out, intentionally symbolic self-representation was a communication to the art therapist, created in the language of the treatment experience. He was ready to work on his impaired self-concept—he characterized it as a pervasive

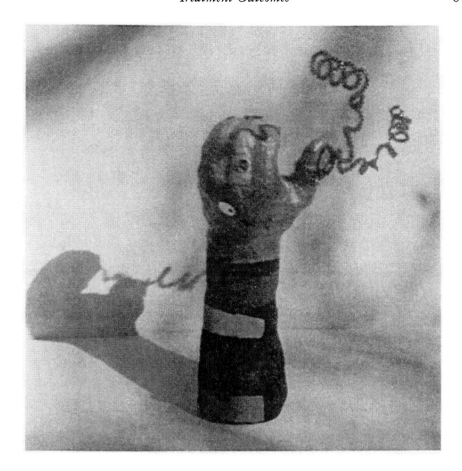

Figure 10. Plaster Sculpture–Hand (Jake).

sense of being "not right, broken, and crazy"—which had for so long sabotaged his academic, social, and emotional growth.

Art therapy proved to be the treatment of choice for this depressed, behavior-disordered youngster. The kinesthetic nature of the art therapy experience provided an opportunity for tension reduction and behavioral focus. The treatment process enabled Jake to gain some distance from his painful and frightening inner world by projecting it onto his artwork, thus making problems and conflicts available for processing. Treatment success brought an acknowledgment from Jake of increased internal locus of control and increased self-esteem, both of which have facilitated Jake's increased willingness to meet serious problems head-on.

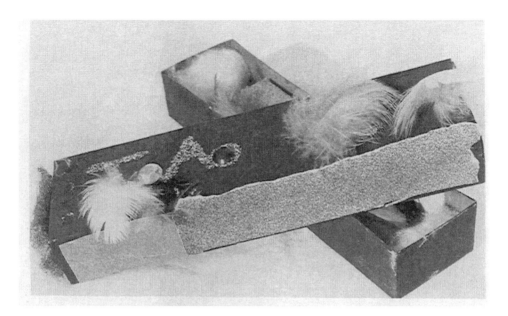

Figure 11. Inside-Outside Box (Jake).

ROSA'S JOURNEY TOWARD BELONGING AND BECOMING REAL

By Linda Jo Pfeiffer

Rosa, a seven-year-old girl of Hispanic ethnic origin, obtained individual art therapy services for more than a year in a self-contained, psychoeducational, elementary program, in a Miami, Florida, public school.

Rosa was born in January 1986. She had entered the program for SED (Severely Emotionally Disturbed) children at age five because of her inability to cope with environmental demands both at home and in school.

Rosa's special education prekindergarten teacher had reported that Rosa had exhibited a combination of aggressive acting-out behavior and severe withdrawal, as well as poor reality functioning, and opposition to authority figures. Psychological testing had supported the judgment. Educational tests had placed Rosa in the average range of intellectual functioning, but her academic performance equalled or surpassed her potential—as gathered from the test results.

Rosa's personal history was complex. When she was 21 months old, she was removed, together with her brother, who was a year older, from the home of her natural mother, owing to deprivation and neglect. Mr. and Mrs. Rodriguez had adopted Rosa, and another member of the Rodriguez family had adopted her brother. Rosa did not know that the son of her aunt and uncle was actually her brother.

When Rosa first arrived at the Rodriguez home, she was delayed in her speech and in her gross and fine motor movements. She did not put words into sentences until age three and one-half. She was also delayed in her toilet training. She had difficulty walking, often stumbling and falling. At age seven, Rosa tended to walk with a stiff, mechanical gait. Her speech was intelligible, but her tone was high-pitched, and her voice had a singsong quality. Her facial features were somewhat pinched and pointed, though she was tall for her age and sturdily built. She was often silly and impulsive in her behavior toward her peers. When interacting with adults, she tended to project a sad or depressed affect. She began taking 25 mg. of Desipramine, an antidepressant, shortly after she started art therapy.

Since Rosa and her brother were privately adopted, there was no state involvement, according to Rosa's mother, who suggested sketchily that there was alcohol or drug preoccupation in the natural home of the children. Rosa and Mrs. Rodriguez had a strong physical resemblance and a strong affective relationship between them.

Rosa lost her status as an only child when Mrs. Rodriguez, at age 35, gave birth to a healthy boy after believing for years that she could not have children. When Mrs. Rodriguez was six months pregnant, she told Rosa that Rosa was adopted.

Rosa had been referred to art therapy to obtain further data about her developmental functioning and as an aid to diagnosis and treatment. Her teachers had observed her tendency to use drawing as a communicative device when she became verbally withdrawn. They were hopeful that Rosa would be able to use art therapy to gain control over her feelings and primitive desires.

The Levick Emotional and Cognitive Art Therapy Assessment (LECATA) was administered to assess Rosa's emotional and cognitive functioning and to develop a treatment plan for her. The six-task assess-

ment yields an emotional and cognitive score related to a child's chronological age. At the time of testing, Rosa's chronological age was 5.11. Her
overall cognitive score was closely aligned with her chronological age; it
was 6.2.

In Task 1 (Figure 12) from the LECATA, her graphic imagery showed
spatial organization, and the objects she had chosen to depict were
recognizable. The beginnings of gender differentiation were apparent in
her drawings.

It was Rosa's emotional score that caused concern. According to the
LECATA, Rosa's emotional score fluctuated from 2½ to 6½ years of
age. A lower level defense mechanism (in the 2½ year old range) found
in Rosa's artwork was incorporation. This was observed in her encapsulated self-portrait, Task 2 (Figure 13). However, Rosa called this contained shape a door, and added a door knob to it suggesting a higher
level defense, simple rationalization. Other instances of the use of lower
level defenses included denial and regression, as found in Tasks 5 and 6
(Figures 15 and 16). A lack of body parts and a notable decline in
graphic abilities were observed. Isolation of affect (in the 6 to 6½ year

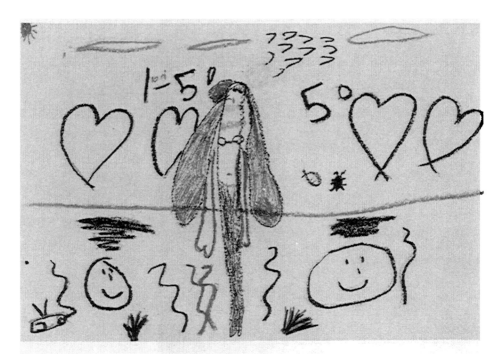

Figure 12. Task 1–Mermaid (Rosa).

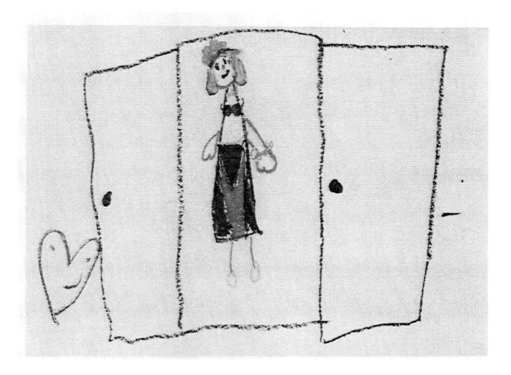

Figure 13. Task 2–Self-Portrait (Rosa).

old normal range) was observed from her use of color in tasks 1 and 2, and her limited use of color in tasks 3 through 6.

The fluctuation in age-appropriate defenses suggested a labile personality that had few personal resources and that regressed easily, using fantasy to escape from perceived stressful situations. The ambivalence and confusion implied in her assessment brought up questions that revolved around Rosa's desire to remain in a more infantile state. Strengths seen in her assessment indicated that in the right environment, Rosa had the potential to use age-appropriate defense mechanisms. Contributing to the results of Rosa's LECATA scores were issues of attachment and separation, which may have been precarious at the time owing to the recent birth of her brother.

Salient features of Rosa's assessment included the degree of magical thinking she engaged in, the tendency toward regression, and the number of unrelated themes she verbally attached to her drawing. During task 5, she talked about a dog that drew, spoke, and told jokes (Figure 15). Rosa had no dog at home. In the family drawing of task 6 (Figure 16), Rosa drew her mother with "ugly hair growing out of the top of her

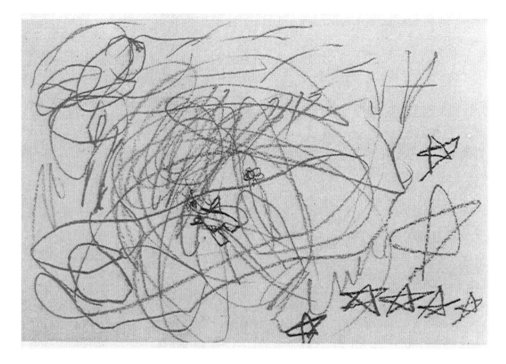

Figure 14. Tasks 3 and 4–A Scribble and a Drawing Created from the Scribble (Rosa).

head, which had to be chopped off and replaced by a flower." She drew her brother and stated that he ate gold. She said little of her father, but he was included in her drawing. Much of the ambivalence and fantasy directed toward her family may have resulted from her learning of her adoption. After the scribble, tasks 3 and 4 (Figure 14), Rosa regressed notably. The theme of her scribble was one of loss and sadness. As the assessment session progressed, it became evident that Rosa was able to keep the boundaries of her fantasy controlled only for a short period of time. She began to draw the number 50 all over her first task (Figure 12), and she added squiggle lines. Rosa stated that in the classroom, earning 50 points was a "first place day."

The results of Rosa's assessment led to the following goals and objectives. Rosa needed to:

1. Increase her reality contact by using art media and associated verbalizations to project real themes and issues.
2. Increase her feelings of self-worth, competency, and pride by

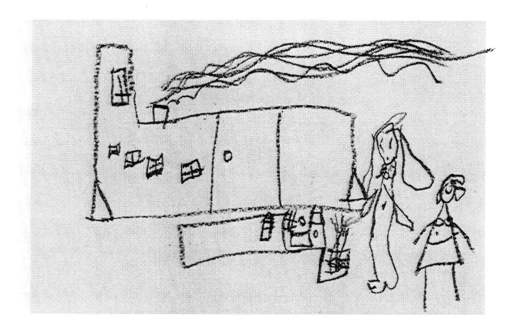

Figure 15. Task 5–Favorite Place (Rosa).

using the art media to increase self-awareness in age-appropriate, productive ways.

3. Increase her ability to identify and express feelings, thoughts, and problems by using art in a communicative fashion to facilitate understanding and resolution.

Rosa enjoyed the art media and used art expressively in individual art therapy sessions, creating satisfying artworks. Initially, she tested limits in the sessions. She appeared to need to know if someone was available to help her control her impulsivity. Without structure, the media would often overwhelm her and she would regress, undoing any product she had completed. This was observed when she spent longer than 20 minutes focused on any one given project. After a period of about a year, Rosa could successfully spend 30 to 40 minutes on a project.

Rosa's behavior vacillated with each art therapy session. Sometimes her shoulders would slump forward, her head would hang down, and eye contact would disappear. She would comply with directives, but would remain quiet, distant, and withdrawn. At other times, Rosa

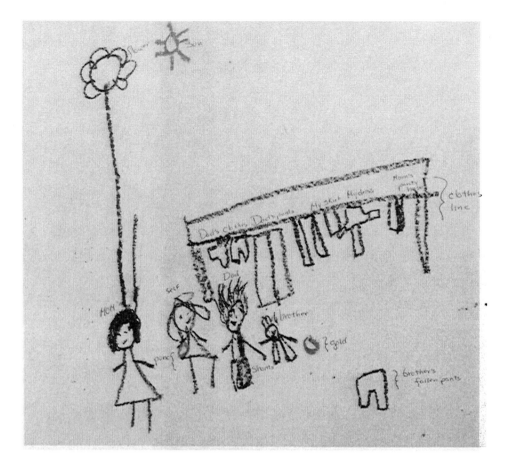

Figure 16. Task 6–Family (Rosa).

would become a delightful child, filled with chatter and little anecdotal recollections of her day. These vacillations could never be tied to environmental situations. Rosa's affect was guided by some internal locus of control, the source of which was unknown to the observer. Because of Rosa's changing spirit, both directive and nondirective art therapy approaches were used.

The consistent themes throughout the year were family and adoption, belonging and not belonging, guilt and fear of rejection. In a particularly revealing set of sessions, Rosa used clay to depict a family of ducks. The scenario played and replayed was of the mother and father duck discarding a dying egg and getting a new one. Was it possible that Rosa feared her parents would replace her with her brother? Was she concerned that they would give her back? The artwork and ensuing discussions opened the way for conversations about adoption and belonging. They also provided a way to increase communication with Rosa's mother about her child's fears and doubts. Her mother, who had carried her baby brother's photograph on both her wristwatch and key chain, was able to see things from Rosa's perspective.

In another session, Rosa drew a picture of herself and then quickly labeled it her brother (Figure 17). She then drew herself in a more attractive, mature fashion. She became confused and stated that sometimes she is herself and sometimes she is her brother. Interestingly, whenever she was asked to depict positive aspects of herself, Rosa responded with a drawing of her family (Figure 18). The degree to which she was unable to focus upon herself alone may be indicative of the separation anxiety associated with poor attachment. Rosa's mother

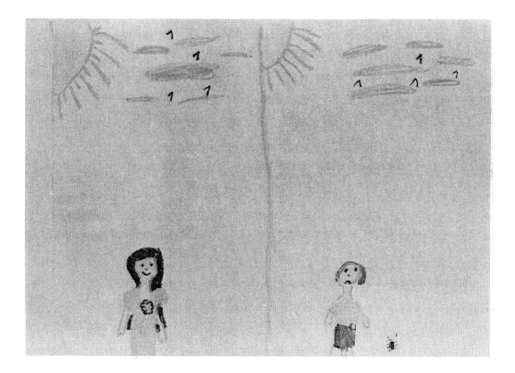

Figure 17. Rosa and Her Brother (Rosa).

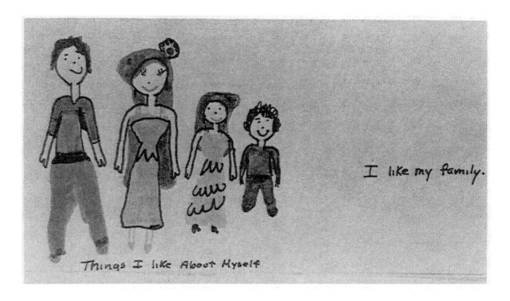

Figure 18. Rosa's Family (Rosa).

often appeared depressed and listless. Was her mother unable to provide the environment for appropriate bonding, or had earlier recollections of neglect and abandonment begun to surface from Rosa's unconscious?

Throughout the past year, one constant image (the Little Mermaid) appeared in Rosa's artwork (Figure 19). Providing Rosa with a safe forum for self-discovery, the Little Mermaid became her heroine, her successful, lovable, and beautiful self. She was able to re-create herself in the perfect image of her dreams. Rosa's underwater sea creature lived in a self-made world where unconditional love reigned supreme (Figure 20). Through the safety of the Little Mermaid, Rosa was able to talk about her true feelings, fears, and wishes. She could encounter problems and find ways to overcome them. Leaving the world of magic fantasy will be a difficult journey for Rosa as she grows and matures.

Art therapy as part of Rosa's educational program is an integral component of her learning. Art therapy has provided her with the consistent support she needs for social and emotional growth as well as for academic achievement.

Rosa continues to receive individual art therapy once a week. If approached from a reality orientation, she becomes evasive and angry. Confronting Rosa with her withdrawal as a way of expressing anger has allowed for increased trust and understanding between Rosa and this

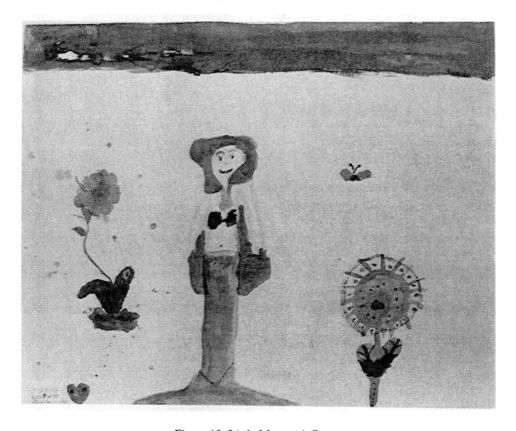

Figure 19. Little Mermaid (Rosa).

therapist. The beginnings of insight, self-awareness, and reflective thought have been observed in recent sessions.

Future art therapy will endeavor to support Rosa's search for an acceptable real self. More body image awareness activities will be provided on a larger scale, allowing for freedom of movement and expression. Following Rosa's lead, adoption issues may direct future art therapy sessions. Graphic expression continues to be her avenue for communication. With support, it may eventually become her personal road to increased reality contact. Meanwhile, Rosa is an avid image-maker, and she states that she is going to be an artist when she grows up.

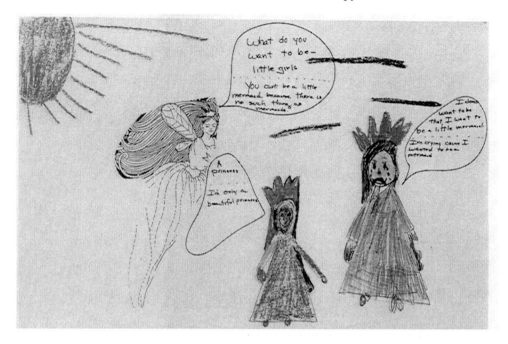

Figure 20. Little Mermaid (Rosa).

Chapter 9

OPERATING CONDITIONS

Standards for such physical needs as the working environment, materials, equipment, and supplies reflect different patterns of availability, deployment, use, consumption, deterioration, repair, and budgetary planning, and operating conditions vary from one school district to another.

My firm conviction is that the treatment space used in art therapy must be appropriate to the task. Every art therapist and student should have convenient access to a soothing treatment setting, one that engenders trust and that spawns a free exchange of comments. The following resources are essential, and schools should provide for them: a separate room that may be used for individual or small group art therapy sessions; locked storage for art supplies and program documentation; art therapy materials, equipment, and supplies; and clerical help to aid in the preparation of art therapy documentation.

ART THERAPY FACILITIES AND THE WORKING ENVIRONMENT

The nature of art therapy is highly confidential, and private space must be maintained. In the Dade County Public schools, the quality of the space varies. The availability of the rooms is dependent on the situations at the individual school sites. Many art therapists have never had the luxury of a private room. They share a room with other school professionals, or travel to classrooms serving youngsters in the back of the room. Some art therapists have had their own rooms, but the facilities have been inadequate—too small and ill-equipped to handle groups and supplies. Other art therapists have been more fortunate, having inherited large, new art studios, fully equipped. Still others, relying on the success they have had in applying their services, have been able to convince their school administrators to assign them suitable space.

Achieving success, in the face of what appear to be observably conflicting goals, calls for considerable energy and dedication on the part of school staff and planners, and necessitates considerable reassurance of captive students. In Bettelheims's opinion (1974), "The environment is an essential part of therapy." The physical environment does affect human behavior, and settings are needed that are congruent with the support goals of the treatment program if the desired results are to be attained.

The physical environment of a treatment facility can, through careful design, provide both a safe and a supportive base for the treatment program: safe in the sense that the area can be built to protect students from hurting themselves or from incurring the violence of others; supportive in the sense that the enclosed area respects the basic human need for privacy, rest, diversion, stimulation, and variety, and assists the staff and the students in the treatment process.

The insecurity connected with a makeshift, changing work site is destabilizing. A permanent and separate room for each art therapist should be the norm—a private counsel-type of room, to ensure confidentiality and to allow for a broad range of equipment, materials, and processes. Time and energy would not have to be wasted then in carrying materials from room to room; nor would feelings of continuity, so important in a therapeutic ambience, be breached; and further, the overall climate would betoken protection from harm, such as the harm that could result from the leaking of innermost feelings and personal data.

Many conditions in the physical environment inhibit a person's sense of comfort and well-being. Elevated stress levels can lead to patterns of disruptive behavior, reduced quality of performance, and general malaise. Stress is a common condition among youngsters experiencing emotional crisis. Because typical classroom hustle-bustle is often stress-inducing, the potential for a difficult treatment session is high. In theory, a high degree of psychic comfort and security would contribute to a positive outlook on a task being performed (Ahrentzen, Jue, Skorpanich and Evans, 1982).

Effective teachers tend to be managers who plan environments that minimize the chances for confusion, distraction, and misbehavior (Brophy, 1983). Nevertheless, since schools are overcrowded, space planning is often not an option. Some students are able to "screen out" ordinary noise and commotion as they work. By reason of motivation or disposition, they are able to focus their attention on the task at hand in spite of nearby disorder. Nonscreeners are students who have difficulty ignoring ordinary visual or auditory phenomena, students who are easily distracted by noise or movement. In the process of trying to overcome the effects of environmental stress—and working hard to cope with emotion—nonscreeners may be sidetracked by distractions, and their attention may wander from the activity at hand.

Over the years, numerous theories have been advanced to describe the impact of a given environment on the behavior of those living and working within it. A number of organizations, including the National Science Foundation, the National Institute of Mental Health, the American Association for the Advancement of Science, and the American Institute of Architects, have sponsored programs to define the relationships between individuals and their environment in specific scientific terms.

The therapeutic environment is part of the basic structure in the treatment and in the relationship between the therapist and the student. Ideal facilities should exemplify the value of a well-designed therapeutic environment, conducive to the creation of artwork; functional, healthful, and aesthetically appropriate. The work center should be organized and suitably equipped for a variety of art media. Furniture should have appropriate seating and large work surfaces, and should include easels, flat-topped tables, stools, and chairs. Lighting should be well placed and sufficiently bright for the artwork. A sink with a trap for grease, clay, and plaster—with adequate counter space for clean up—should be accessible for projects involving water, and should be large enough and deep enough to handle buckets and other materials. The work space should be large enough and planned for sufficient flexibility to permit varied individual and group activities. Facilities for disabled students should insure ease of movement for wheelchairs, sink and work surfaces that are adapted in height, organization sensible to the blind, and safety.

The art therapist's station should provide adequately for personal effects, desk work, preparation of session materials, and lockable storage. There should be appropriate display space—a chalkboard and tackboard within the room, display areas planned throughout the school, and a system for hanging and attaching work to ceilings and walls. An adequate number of electrical outlets should be conveniently placed, and should provide sufficient power for special equipment needs. The acoustical treatment should minimize the noise level and help to maintain privacy. Ventilation should be adequate to exhaust dust, odors, and fumes. Floor surfaces should be easily cleanable, and should have damage-resistant finishes.

A kiln must be appropriately placed within the school to conform to building and electrical safety codes. Shelving must provide for adequate storage of papers and other supplies, and space and equipment must be adequate for drying wet products. Storage for student works of art must also be adequate.

Clerical support for the preparation of art therapy documentation can enhance the ease with which the reporting process is achieved. If clerical support is available, art therapists should work with the administrative offices to carry out procedures for the word processing of art therapy documentation. If computers are available, art therapists should have access to them for the preparation of their written documentation. All art therapy reports should be typed, as assessments and progress reports become part of the permanent record in a student's file, and must be understandable.

MATERIALS, EQUIPMENT, AND SUPPLIES

The variety and complexity of art forms, media, and artistic expression do not make it possible to specify all the essentials requisite for the educational process, art products, management, and budget, but the quality of the materials and equipment used and the nature of the background experiences are important determiners of outcomes in a meaningful art therapy program. Art therapists need to use high quality materials. If the quality of the art materials is low, the artistic ability required may have to be high. Also, a variety of materials must be available if students are to experience a range of art expressions.

Whatever the purchasing of supplies involves, the art therapy staff of a school or district should provide input in the specification of the standards for art materials, equipment, and resources that will be consumed through the practice of art therapy. This is a competency to be expected and respected.

Materials and equipment should allow for a comprehensive art therapy program that can cover a broad range of methods, such as painting, drawing, printmaking, collage, sculpture, photography, crafts, ceramics, fiber arts, jewelry, and wood. The personal background experience and philosophical orientation of each art therapist should contribute to the selection of the materials and artistic direction for every session. A kiln and paper cutter should be available, and office supplies needed for the preparation of session documentation should be readily at hand.

BUDGET

It is difficult to identify an objective concept for the reasonable cost of an equipment and materials budget. An adequate budget must promote a consistent program of supply, maintenance, and improvement. A budget for art therapy must be distinct in a school's budget allocation. It should have sufficient funds to provide for required expenditures on consumable materials, student and staff resource materials (books, professional journals and publications, media materials), and new replacement and equipment repair materials and supplies. Additional budgetary expenditures that would enhance an art therapy program would involve the production of documents that communicate information about a program (handouts and brochures), inservice education, and other support or professional development. If available, a reserve fund could provide incentive for research, special projects, conferences, scholarships, and educational travel. Budgets for art therapy should be commensurate with budgets provided for all other areas of the school program. Budgetary planning should assume the increases in cost per student and should be adjusted for rates of inflation.

A well-organized budget could be made more or less routine at every school site that sustains art therapy. An equitable distribution of funds would support both therapist and student morale, and would enable a district or school to plan and assess a successful art therapy program.

Chapter 10

COLLABORATION WITH PARENTS AND WITH SCHOOL AND AGENCY PROFESSIONALS

Collaboration is an important aspect of the relationships formed by school art therapists. As indicated in previous chapters, art therapists carry the responsibility for planning and implementing a variety of services for students with special needs. Although they develop the comprehensive programs for such students, the challenge cannot be fully met without assistance and support from other professionals—in the school system and in community agencies—and from parents and the community. The alliances the school art therapists form with others are essential for the effective delivery of the broad spectrum of services expected in a comprehensive school art therapy program.

Professionals who work in community agencies can be especially helpful to school art therapists. Their understanding of the professional roles and functions of school art therapists can aid considerably in establishing "helping" services for students and in forming cooperative consulting relationships with the members of all school treatment teams.

This chapter is about the working relationships that school art therapists maintain with individuals, parents and guardians, professionals, and agencies.

PARENTS AND GUARDIANS

Parental involvement is a vital ingredient of successful school art therapy at all levels of practice. School art therapists must make every effort to establish lines of communication with the home, and must invite parents and guardians to join in planning and carrying out the goals for their children.

It is incumbent upon all helping professionals within schools to form cooperative working relationships with parents and guardians, especially

86

for the selection and implementation of strategies. Involvement will support the efforts made not only by the art therapists but by the entire school treatment team.

The first step in the process is to learn about the families served by the schools and to determine the needs of the parents and guardians by assessing the roles they expect to play in the treatment of their children. The relationships the art therapists establish with the parents and guardians may be an important predictor of success in the individual and small group counseling sessions students attend. It is particularly so for youngsters with special emotional needs who have little control over their home environments and the situations that influence their lives.

By collaborating with parents and guardians, school art therapists create the avenue through which they provide their direct services and their indirect assistance. Parents and guardians obviously have a tremendous impact on the choices that children make regarding school performance, career direction, friendships, and other important facets of their development. By consulting with the parents and guardians, school art therapists are better able to design support networks and channels of communication that can complement the goals and objectives of the therapy they provide, and parents and guardians are better able to contribute to the development of the strategies that will nurture positive adult-child relationships at home.

Art therapists frequently contact parents about student progress in art therapy, and consult about ways to support the children's social/emotional development at home. Art therapists who believe that facilitative relationships are essential for improving home-school communications contribute considerably to the establishment of mutual respect between parents and teachers. Relationships such as these can help the children to develop to their fullest potential.

Art therapists also provide direct services for parents and guardians through educational programs. Parenting is a challenging role for which few are prepared in any formal sense. Most people have learned parenting skills by adapting a model exercised by their own parents. Unfortunately, the behaviors learned are not always conducive to the healthy development of children. To assist in the parenting process, school art therapists can establish support groups and lead the parent education programs. When possible, family art therapy sessions can be held, and can prove to be beneficial in the treatment of family issues. All of these forums are designed to help parents exchange ideas about what works with their children and in their families, and help in the utilization of collective knowledge in choosing appropriate alternatives to current situations.

Parent work schedules must be arranged to accommodate this type of service. To fit their work schedules, parent groups usually meet at night, but they also arrange to attend meetings during the day. Art therapists scheduling parent groups during the day should seek input from their principals to examine the ramifications of using school time to assist the parents. If positive parenting skills equate to increased learning and participation of the students in school, art therapists should be able to convince principals and teachers of the importance of daytime activities.

Few students develop at optimal levels without support and encouragement from their parents and guardians. Through direct contact, art therapists can provide current information, needed parenting skills, clarification of family issues, and essential problem-solving services. Art therapists who work with parents and guardians can make certain that schools and families move in the same direction and have similar goals for the students. To verify the parallel movement, art therapists need to consult and collaborate with the teachers in addition to the school treatment teams.

SCHOOLS

Students with special needs often have conditions that so interfere with their learning processes that special services—like art therapy— have to be provided. The services become clinical complements to the instructional program. The instruction and its related support services are interwoven to form an integrated unit that will respond to the specific needs of the affected children. A well-coordinated and comprehensive plan is necessary to achieve the goal. For each student, a collaborative process is initiated that utilizes the expertise of the entire group—teacher, clinicians, school administrators, other support personnel, art therapist, and parents. The collaborative process—the core element of success, both for the students and the program—is referred to as multidisciplinary program implementation. Neither the instructional component nor the art therapy component can stand alone. Intertwined, however, they contribute to the positive outcomes toward which a team approach and professional expertise lead. Joint face-to-face planning sessions, meetings with parents, monitoring, and periodic reviews, together with ongoing mutual feedback between staff members who work with given students, tie loose ends together.

The network of information exchange is needed to allow both clinical and instructional staff to expand their knowledge of the individual student's functioning and to consider the ways in which the services they render can complement the targeted areas or intervention strategies used by the other team members. This ongoing collaborative cycle of planning, implementation, and feedback between instructional staff, clinical support staff, and parents is what gives the students the comprehensive therapeutic educational approach they require.

Forums for planning and implementation strategies may include case conferences and departmental meetings at which the student cases or programming strategies are addressed. When a clear division of roles and responsibilities for a given program has been established, the team members can proceed with ease. When there is no clear leadership, the task is more difficult. The program director or primary clinician may have the responsibility for providing the leadership necessary to maintain the team approach, or the art therapist may have to maintain a direct approach and carry out his/her own roles and responsibilities for the best art therapy job possible.

In the early years of the Dade County program, acceptance of art therapy and art therapists did not come readily. Art therapy service designed to support the school psychologist or the art teacher was often perceived as a substitute service. It took years of hard work among clinical members of the school staff and art teachers to establish the clear role played by art therapy. It is still difficult to implement art therapy in schools that have had no prior experience with it. It is also difficult to delineate the distinctions between the art therapy procedures and the procedures of art teachers and school psychologists for upper level management and for school administrators who have had no prior knowledge of art therapy.

Three key factors contributed to the acceptance of art therapy methods by other clinical members of the school staff and by art teachers at the Dade County schools:

1. Art therapists showed positive outcomes when their roles and responsibilities were carried out independently. Their professional confidence and their maintenance of a clear and knowledgeable attitude relative to the work being accomplished paralleled the results needed in each situation.

2. In presentations on art therapy at such forums as inservice programs and case conferences for selected audiences of school psychologists and art teachers, the art therapists were able to share the benefits that had been derived from the art therapy approach.

3. The art therapists gave assistance to the personnel with whom they worked. This included the school principal, the teachers, and the other clinicians.

The old concept of "one hand washing the other" benefited both parties and assisted in building a team. The work of the art therapists as facilitators—persons whose job it is to provide assistance, information, training, and support—was crucial in furthering the collaborative school improvement efforts. When the art therapists were perceived as friendly and helpful individuals, and successful performers in cases that other professionals could not manage, the barriers to working relationships fell.

The key to achieving success in all outcomes was consistency. It was not enough to have a positive attitude one day and not the next. It was not enough to provide one presentation. There had to be a series of planned efforts to help educate colleagues. A collaborative process that was built upon respect for each professional's role, responsibilities, and skills not only enhanced the services provided to each student but benefited the whole program.

A team approach surfaced involving regular meetings in which the staff members shared information, updated cases, and assigned responsibilities that would avoid the duplication of services. They also focused on specific cases to ensure that students were receiving appropriate services from the school and that referrals to community resources were adequately pursued and monitored.

Effective collaboration among staff members in schools begins with mutual understanding and respect for separate roles, with regard for individual areas of expertise. In situations where this respect and regard are not achieved, services for students are not well coordinated, and students' needs are inadequately addressed.

In today's schools, students, parents, and teachers are faced with challenges that call for services from a variety of professionals. The differences of purpose and training in the professional applications of each specialization are apparent. Adequate coordination and timely collaboration make it possible to provide appropriate and effective services for all concerned. A harmonious whole provides a sense of fulfillment—a feeling of integration of duties—rather than a sense of infringement on categorical responsibility. Consider the term "related school personnel," which may include the following staff members, all of whose roles are different from those of an art therapist and different from those of each other, but all of whom have a basic and specialized background in psychology. It becomes incumbent upon each of them to tailor their individual focus and knowledge to fit a supererogatory intent. For example:

Counselor:	Provides individual and group academic and vocational counseling; academic testing, administration, and interpretation; course scheduling; personal counseling; and consultation with teachers, parents, and community sources to identify student academic or vocational needs and to select appropriate services.
School Psychologist:	Engages in psychological and psychoeducational assessment and evaluation measures to provide assistance in school placement; and in the selection of services to assist youngsters in benefiting from education; also, in inservice training, parent counseling, program planning and evaluation, and parent education.
Social Worker:	Proceeds with facilitation and monitoring of the relationship between home and school, often resulting in case management; and with coordination between home and school to ensure communication and follow-through to help meet student needs.
Special Education Teacher:	Gives instruction to children and adolescents who require special education services through adapted curriculums, to meet individual student needs; evaluates students, plans and carries out educational goals and objectives as indicated on a student's Individualized Education Plan (IEP).

They all join forces to achieve the given end. They use their backgrounds in psychology to perform their assigned duties and to extend themselves to reach a higher, more encompassing measure of achievement.

PRINCIPALS/SCHOOL ADMINISTRATORS

Schools and special programs are managed by administrators trained in educational administration, curriculum, law, and other aspects of school governance. These administrators are responsible for everything that goes on in a school building: all programs and services. Therefore, every service and activity scheduled by school art therapists is directly or indirectly supervised by a school principal. This responsibility makes it essential for school principals and school art therapists to collaborate on the activities of the art therapy program—including selection of major goals and objectives, roles and responsibilities, student progress, special events, and all the other activities that are part of a comprehensive school art therapy program. A collaborative relationship with the school principal should be an ongoing effort. Art therapists should share program planning activities with their principals, and, at the same time, should be ready to inform other pertinent school administrators of the issues and concerns that affect student development.

Many activities planned by art therapists have a schoolwide focus to meet the needs of a broad spectrum of students, parents, and teachers. In determining goals and strategies for these schoolwide events, art therapists have to collaborate with the principals and other administrators to be sure of the feasibility and appropriateness of the activities. Since principals have knowledge of local policies, financial limitations, and other restrictions that guide the selection and implementation of the activities and events planned by a school, established working relationships with school principals can keep school art therapists fully informed about the parameters within which their programs and services are required to operate.

When sharing information with school principals and other administrators, art therapists should be careful to follow ethical standards and legal guidelines regarding confidential materials and privileged communications. Art therapists frequently receive confidential information in helping-relationships with students, and this information must remain private unless there is imminent danger to others.

COMMUNITY AGENCIES AND SERVICES

At times, the emotional and personal concerns raised by students with art therapists and the treatment team require in-depth interventions. While art therapists and other members of the treatment team are competent to offer interventions, the degree of student need and the staff time, schedules, and other factors associated with school art therapy services make it more appropriate to refer students and families to mental health settings, including hospitals, agencies, and clinically-oriented placements, as well as to private practitioners, rather than to the school treatment team. Collaboration between an outside facility and the art therapist and treatment team are essential because while students are receiving treatment at the outside facility, they usually remain in school and continue their contacts with the art therapist. If the students are hospitalized or are receiving services at a residential setting, the helping relationship will be resumed upon their return to school.

Chapter 11

ENHANCING THE
PROFESSIONAL DEVELOPMENT
OF A SCHOOL ART THERAPIST

Professional development activities for art therapists and other pertinent school personnel should be regularly implemented to be sure they
are versed in the technical and affective aspects of treatment. Comprehensive professional development not only provides a professional forum
for interchange, but allows staff members to expand their knowledge
and to grow. At the same time, professional development serves as a
highly effective public relations tool because it promotes awareness of the
field of art therapy and, by example, demonstrates the ongoing benefits
that accrue to individual youngsters from its application.

Two aspects of professional growth and skill development are evident
in a comprehensive program: (1) inservice training—sessions designed
for art therapists; sessions provided by staff art therapists for school
personnel; and other professional sessions, such as national, state, and
local conferences and seminars, and (2) program evaluation procedures.

INSERVICE TRAINING

Staff development sessions designed for art therapists provide them
with information on art therapy strategies and techniques, and with
technical information related to the treatment of youngsters with special
needs. The sessions are intended to update the knowledge and expertise
of the staff art therapists.

Enhancement sessions were most useful in the early years of the Dade
County program. There were no courses to update knowledge and skills.
Local university level art therapy programs were nonexistent. The Dade
County Public Schools Art Therapy Department found it necessary to
plan a series of sessions on a variety of topics based on staff interest. Some
sessions were presented by clinicians from local hospitals and agencies,

or by nationally known art therapists who were contracted for the occasion; other sessions were presented by the staff art therapists themselves. Among the topics discussed were Art Therapy and Child Abuse, Multiple Personalities and the Art Therapy Process, Family Art Psychotherapy, and Multicultural Aspects of Art Therapy.

The art therapists also learned from their own processing and review of individual student cases and from the exploration of general topics of interest. In addition, small group/peer supervision sessions were useful in promoting awareness of treatment approaches.

When reviewing student cases, the following areas should be addressed:

1. Highlights of clinical history
2. Clinical observations
3. Art tasks that are implemented
4. Findings (e.g., cognitive and emotional development, themes, conflicts, strengths)
5. Recommendations for other types of support services (e.g., family therapy, speech therapy, group therapy)
6. Art therapy goals and objectives

Peer group meetings can be conducted in the afternoons when the students leave school. Supplementary activities that may be planned include book reviews, hands-on experiences, and special guest presentations by mental health personnel.

Observations of fellow art therapists in the school district or in other settings can also enhance professional service delivery considerably. They can, for example, serve to update art therapy techniques and strategies. Site visits should be planned with the approval of the school administration, and should incorporate guidelines such as:

1. Meet all staff and program administrators.
2. Observe sessions.
3. Read program documentation reports.
4. Engage in a dialogue on sessions observed.
5. Discuss art therapy techniques and strategies, and the materials used with various students.
6. Discuss methods used for storing artwork and supplies.

Staff development sessions provided by art therapists for school personnel are designed to promote an understanding of art therapy practices and student progress. Such sessions are important for eliminating barriers to staff communication and for assisting staff members in understanding the art therapy techniques and strategies that may be adapted to their work and that can assist them in understanding students with special needs. Topics can be wide-ranging: e.g., introduction to art therapy; art therapy assessment; developing an awareness of the creative process and its relation to child development; what children are expressing through their art; art therapy principles for the classroom teacher; normal developmental benchmarks and warning signals in children's artwork; applications of media techniques to spur student development; expressive group art therapy; art therapy applications for such specific diagnostic groups as adolescents or dually-diagnosed individuals; chemical dependency; family treatment and abuse; and the presentation of individual student cases. Sessions can include didactic as well as experiential activities.

The scheduling time of sessions conducted by art therapists for school personnel, whether they are to be brief inservice sessions or sessions planned for a full day, can be arranged. Some schools have arranged for training days when there were no students present in school. Lack of time or difficulty in finding time should not prevent an art therapist from scheduling such sessions. They are, by far, the most important aspect of public relations, and merit high priority on an art therapist's "do" list.

Selected conferences and workshops—national, state, and local—and professional seminars offered in conjunction with universities, colleges, hospitals, and agencies are designed to promote an art therapist's professional competencies. Individual school programs may have a budget to help cover the expenses of registration and travel fees. If not, art therapists may have to incur the expenses themselves. Nevertheless, by attending selected sessions they can enhance their understanding of practices and approaches to treatment. Art therapists should consult with administrators about obtaining permission to attend these sessions, as attendance may entail leaving a school site and on-site job responsibilities.

The practice of school art therapy has undergone, and will continue to undergo, significant changes as new knowledge and technological advances are introduced. The development of new intervention techniques, assessment procedures, and computerized assistance will require practitioners to keep abreast of innovations, as well as to obtain appropriate professional education and training in specific areas. All school art therapists should participate in the activities designed to help them continue, enhance, and upgrade their professional training and skills. Membership in professional organizations; the reading of professional journals and books; discussions with colleagues on professional issues; attendance at professional workshops, seminars, and conferences; and the presentations they conduct on their own programs and services are all integral to a school art therapist's overall and continuing professional development.

PROGRAM EVALUATION PROCEDURES

A comprehensive system of standardized procedures and a variety of instruments are used in assessing the performance of all school art therapists. A Program Support Checklist, a version of which appears as Appendix J, is a useful "guide," which any art therapist who wishes to stay on track can consult.

The following assumptions exist with regard to program evaluation:

1. Quality education can be achieved through a concerted effort by all educational staff members who are accountable for the quality of education in a school district.
2. Educational staff members are competent professionals desirous of maintaining a continuous pattern of professional growth and skill development.
3. School administrators are charged with the responsibility for instructional program management/evaluations.
4. Enhancement of professional skills is a key responsibility of the school district's administrative and support staff.
5. Specific kinds of professional behavior are essential to meaningful education.

Chapter 12

PUBLIC RELATIONS

The Art Therapy Program of the Dade County Public Schools has steadily acquired supporters since 1979, not only within the student body, but among school staff, parents, and other concerned members of the Dade County school district. Through expansion and popularity, it has become a significant part of student services. It has aroused attention nationally, and a number of efforts have been made to replicate program features.

Proponents of art therapy in other communities need to do considerable advance planning and research, and it is advisable that they start the work on a small scale in order to overcome resistance; then, they can go on and tailor the program to local needs and facilities.

Public relations is an important aid in the effort to get such a program off the ground. Effective public relations action can energize interest. However, it takes time to reach the point at which acceptance is assured, and initiators should not lose hope. They must continue their efforts at all stages of the activity if they wish to be successful.

Art therapists need to take the lead in demonstrating the value of art therapy to the public. Art therapists need to engage in public relations, knowing that the public is learning to believe in art therapy, and that it makes a difference in the way people understand themselves and each other—and how they accept responsibility for their lives. In art therapy, people learn how they can change faulty behavior—they learn to adjust their attitudes gradually, until they can cope with the conditions that have led to their unproductive manifestations.

We know it is necessary to build a confident, competent, cooperative, concerned society, a society that appreciates individuals who are creative and sensitive to the beauties and values of a good life. We must find ways to help children grow into productive adults, competent and cooperative because they respect themselves. We must lift the spirits of dejected students, and raise the potential of all our citizens. By helping children, through art therapy, to better understand themselves and life, we can give them a chance to succeed in life. We must find ways to communicate this message to parents, to administrators, to community leaders, and to taxpayers (Bush, 1995).

Part of being a successful art therapist is taking personal responsibility for public relations. No one is going to promote art therapy unless art therapists do. If art therapy is to be a part of education and a strong force for good in our society, art therapists must learn to make society actively aware of its value. They must emphasize its importance to the growth and well-being of every child, and its necessity in a society that values individuality and the quality of life.

Public relations will be effective in the field of art therapy if art therapists take an active role in school and community affairs: in committees, service organizations, and cultural functions. Those who are not joiners can take advantage of their contacts with friends, students, neighbors, and acquaintances, to speak out for art therapy. I say to art therapists: Take the initiative—popularize art therapy in any way you can!

Who are the people you want to reach through public relations? Everyone! For example:

- The school board member who would rather hire drug counselors for troubled children—why hire art therapists when the system has already cut back on art teachers?
- The administrator who has cut the budget—art therapy is not really an essential requirement.
- The taxpayer who wants to cut out all the frills—reading, math, and science are what will prepare youngsters for the real world.
- The citizen who believes that helping children can only be accomplished by the school psychologist.
- The teacher who says that her students are not "talented" in art—so why have art therapy?

All of these responses reveal a gross misunderstanding of what art therapy is all about. Art therapists must reach out! They must define their audiences! They must communicate with those with whom they already have contact—and find ways to become involved with the others! Their audiences must be: Parents, teachers, students, school administrators, school board members, political leaders, business people, news media personnel, and community leaders.

I believe that empathy is a key to successful public relations. People must be good listeners. They need to find out what other persons are thinking and feeling about how art therapy can help. Do you know what your local school board members or school administrators think of art therapy? Have any of them ever known an art therapist? Have art therapists ever shown them the value of art therapy for general education?

Ask yourself: Is there a chance that somewhere in between all the budgets and meetings, the administrator may believe—or can believe—in the importance of achieving improved academic functioning through a nontraditional modality such as art therapy? Has an art therapist ever asked an administrator to speak out on the importance of art therapy?

Whether a new art therapy program is about to be started, or whether a program is already in effect, I believe that all art therapists have two major forces to overcome through ongoing public relations: apathy and attitudes.

Apathy

There are always those who do not care . . . about the arts, mental health, a misunderstood and nontraditional area such as art therapy. Since they do not care, they will not be concerned if art therapy never makes an entrance into an educational program.

To combat apathy, art therapists must teach others what art therapy is and why it is important. How? Through public relations:

- Through a long, continual program of presentations, meetings, classes, workshops, displays, and promotions, and through involvement with others.
- Through case studies on how art therapy has helped youngsters in crisis achieve success.
- Through consistent emphasis on the self-understanding that takes place in the art therapy treatment room.

People need to see art therapy in action. They can experience it through exhibits, on-site demonstrations, videos, and participation workshops. Constant emphasis should be placed on the values of art therapy—through newspapers, signs, posters, talks, television and radio appearances, letters, and everyday conversations.

Art therapists can involve others in helping to promote the field. How?

- By soliciting help with exhibits and programs.
- By inviting individuals to write or speak about art.

- By inviting individuals to write or speak about art therapy.
- By forming lay committees to help promote art therapy.

Attitudes

Some people are not interested in serving the mental health needs of students in the schools. Others have definite ideas on the subject, but their ideas are inadequate or misleading. Some of the major misconceptions are:

- Art therapy is special education art, an activity for disabled children.
- Art therapy is not a real therapy.
- Since school budgets are in crisis, art therapy cannot be considered.
- Art therapy is best suited to very young children.
- Diagnosis and assessment should only be undertaken by psychiatrists and psychologists.
- The school psychologist and the counselor can make more progress in treating troubled children than can an art therapist.
- Families become more involved in their youngster's treatment when a psychiatrist or social worker is involved—not an art therapist.
- Anyone with art training and an interest in special populations can do art therapy.
- There are too many other problems in schools today—drugs, teen pregnancy, and physical violence—art therapy cannot begin to address these problems.
- The school district has no licensure/personnel certification for art therapists, so there is no structure for hiring them.

Art therapists must be aware of and must understand misconceptions in order to counteract them.

PUBLIC RELATIONS IN ACTION

Art therapists in the Dade County Public Schools engage in "public relations" activities on an ongoing basis. Let me share some of the occasions with you.

Faculty Workshops

Inservice sessions on the processes and effects of art therapy are arranged for teachers at each school. The teachers receive an overview of the philosophy behind art therapy applications, and diagnostic and therapeutic theories. Presentations are made of the artwork done by their students in art therapy. Hands-on experiences are also provided the teachers to emphasize particular processes. Hands-on experiences literally bring the key points home to them. Drawing time turns out to be a calming influence, and a process of self-actualization stemming from the verbal associations individual teachers make with what they have drawn. Group members appear to be more at ease after the sessions, and they support their newly evoked interest in art therapy with positive remarks. They are impressed enough with the outcome to make requests of their departments for the integration of art therapy strategies.

Teamwork

My effort to meet with the school counselor as often as possible on the day I spend at a school has proven to be an effective commitment on my part. At our school, the counselor asked me to review several drawings for symbolic interpretation of a troubled adolescent. The student's parents were in the process of getting a divorce, and the student's inner turmoil was manifesting itself in behavioral problems at school.

I recommended art experiences that the counselor could try—for example, the making of small clay figures, representing a family. The counselor could use the figures to role-play with the student. Together they could work through some family troubles and how best to deal with them. I suggested that the counselor assume a noticeable attitude of support to help the boy master his feelings about the divorce.

I also scheduled the boy for an art therapy assessment. Even though the art therapy schedule was full, I arranged the assessment to make sure the counselor had credible feedback. The shared results were positively received. The counselor helped the student to deal with some of his problems, but the counselor was also helped to understand him better. The teamwork brought professional appreciation to an art therapist for her services.

Community

A teacher's sixth grade class of emotionally disturbed students was designing a mural on the wall of the physical education equipment building. Another teacher's class was painting a mural on the wall outside of its classroom. This was all part of a school beautification project to promote the school's existence in the community and to help enhance esteem for the students. It was also an opportunity for the students to attract the attention of other students and teachers in the school and to reach out to the general community.

Time was arranged in my art therapy schedule to provide leadership for this activity on a weekly basis. In between, the teachers handled the painting. The local newspapers were invited to publicize the activity so the community would see that through the medium of art, these troubled youngsters could have their behavior redirected, and could then do something positive for their community. Local dignitaries were invited to a special "opening" to hear accounts of the painting experiences. The project was well-received, and recognition by the local community helped the students to feel proud of their accomplishments.

Each of these cases demonstrates that empathy is the key to a successful art therapy program, and the cornerstone of public relations. Helping our contacts to understand the benefits derived from art therapy helps us all to sell the program. The quality of the program is its own best publicity.

PUBLIC RELATIONS STRATEGIES FOR INITIATING AND CARRYING OUT AN ART THERAPY PROGRAM

Every art therapist in the local area should be involved in general public relations at the community level. Public relations efforts can facilitate administration, prevent misinformation from spreading, generate interest in art therapy, and assist in promoting the accomplishments of students and staff. Scheduling time to initiate a public relations campaign is not only an important step in helping to get an art therapy program started, but in insuring the program's continuance. There are many ways to accomplish the varying tasks imposed by the requirements of public relations. A major responsibility is keeping the program on track and effective.

Perhaps the most difficult job in starting a new program, activity, or service is reaching and influencing individuals who make decisions about education in the community. The individuals to reach include legislators, school board members, special committee members, principals, and various school administrators.

School administrators who are in a position to initiate art therapy services are in such departments as Exceptional Student Education (supervisors for various exceptionalities: e.g., the emotionally disturbed;

the director in charge of all exceptionalities), Guidance and Counseling, Art Education, School Psychology, and Alternative Education. Efforts should be made to contact them because in most instances they will be the decision-makers.

Messages to demonstrate the value of art therapy can be delivered at meetings. Meetings can take place with one administrator or several administrators. If convinced of the value of art therapy, administrators can be a significant force. They are usually sincerely concerned with the well-being of their departments, and can exert a strong influence on both public opinion and educational opinion.

The initial meeting should be brief, simply to let individuals know why art therapy is important in the fulfillment of every child's potential as a person, and to listen to the ideas that are expressed. After this contact, an occasional personal memo or letter should be sent, informing individuals of art therapy developments that are significant for the community. The art therapists must keep these individuals informed on issues, on what is being done, and on how they can give support and encouragement. Ask for advice, opinions, and suggestions. Let the individuals help. Always put yourself in their place and respect their positions, responsibilities, and busy schedules. Always express appreciation for support, help, advice, or participation.

One meeting may not be enough to get a program started—it may take several meetings with key decision-makers to put across the full value of art therapy. Workshops with slide commentaries and visual examples that demonstrate treatment outcomes, presented over and over again, may help to nail down a point. It may take only one key administrator to make the difference—one who believes in change and growth and who has the foresight to try out new educational strategies, as well as the ability to sway other colleagues to the advantages attendant upon a new approach.

At a future meeting, you might present a statement of purpose; a definition of art therapy; a brief overview of an art therapist's training background; mini cases with artwork to demonstrate treatment outcomes; an overview of how art therapy can fit into an educational program; and funding strategies.

The area of funding will no doubt be the hardest to demonstrate since that is very often an obstacle to the initiation of new educational approaches. For disabled students, e.g., those identified as emotionally disturbed and needing special educational services to benefit from the regular educational program, there are monies that can be designated for art therapy through IDEA (Individuals With Disabilities Education Act). Other funding areas might also include nondisabled students and might include grant sources and locally generated monies that are earmarked for particular programs.

Many additional resources may need to be targeted:

- There are grants designed to promote educational endeavors.
- Businesses and industries may often contribute, participate in, and invest in services. Seek them for consultation and funding purposes.
- Pilot a model program for a limited time period, e.g., a year, to demonstrate effectiveness.
- Work through community agencies or in private practice for contracted part-time services with a school or school district.
- Obtain full-time employment as a related service professional, e.g., an art educator, a mental health professional, implementing specifically assigned duties for part of the day and art therapy for another part of the day. Effective promotion of art therapy may eventually make the art therapy service a full-time assignment.
- Make arrangements to provide services for individual students who need art therapy and to provide inservice education for staff personnel.

You may find that any one of the above approaches will suit your purpose, or be convinced that a combination of approaches will work better in an individual school or school district.

Ongoing Promotional Efforts

Once a service is initiated, promotion cannot stop, as the best publicity is the success of an ongoing program. A planned program of public relations needs to be developed and maintained. Steps that will prove useful are:

Initiate a series of staff development workshops that target such audiences as teachers, administrators, counselors, and psychologists, and that demonstrate how art therapy can help the students.

Send out invitations to parents. Invite them to participate in workshops on why art therapy is important, on the creative process and child development, and on the cognitive and emotional development of children through art.

Prepare visual displays, such as educational art therapy exhibits, accompanied by narratives explaining the art activity and the emotional process that took place, resulting in the particular product. Set up the displays in schools, banks, airports, the city hall, businesses, and the school administration offices.

Facilitate panel presentations, forums, and seminars conducted by key community members at which art therapists will address particular topics. For example, a seminar led by a local college professor or dignitary might deal with the creative process and mental health. An art therapist could describe a case history in which a bad imprint made on a child's mind is gradually resolved as a result of sound art therapy treatment.

Arrange for visual presentations—videotapes, slides, posters, brochures, flyers—that explain aspects of art therapy.

On occasion, let interested professionals and students in training benefit from observing an art therapy session. Approval should first be obtained from the school administrator, and the proper release forms must be on file. The activity will promote viewer understanding of the approach, format, and implementation strategies being used. The art therapist may provide the following materials to the visitors, to enhance the quality of their observations: the student artwork folder or selected artworks, neatly organized for viewing; the weekly art therapy schedule; goals and objectives; the assessment report; the treatment plan; and other available support materials that may be related to a student, as well as requested materials. Handouts and brochures on art therapy services will enhance and promote the observation.

Presentation of Student Cases and Participation at Case Conferences

Case conferences are designed to promote awareness of student progress. There may or may not be a structure for a case conference in the educational program. This varies from school district to school district. An art therapist may want to develop a procedure for a case conference if none exists, or may want to make presentations on particular students on an ongoing basis. The following format lends itself to the sharing of information on student cases:

1. Brief description of setting and location of art therapy service
2. Identification of student and date of birth
3. Summary of data from the record
   admission notes
   diagnosis
   psychological evaluation
   personal history
   family history
4. Referral to art therapy
   reason for referral
   art therapy assessment results
   art therapy goals
5. Description of student
   physical characteristics
   style and manner
   attitude toward art therapy
6. Brief description of art therapy situation
   space
   materials
   number and duration of sessions
   individual or group setting
   approach and style in art therapy
7. Sessions and artwork presentations
   Describe what you think happened therapeutically in the session (relationship and important issues dealt with); questions in your mind; interpretations; relevant theoretical material; important conversations; problems that occurred and what you might have done differently; what you plan to do to help move the therapy along; what you learned from this experience.

OTHER STRATEGIES TO ENHANCE PUBLIC RELATIONS IN A SCHOOL PROGRAM

The following procedures are designed to enhance the relationships between school personnel and students within schools. Proper consent forms must be on file if student information is shared.

1. Display selected student artwork in the school. First, negotiate space with the school principal. Then, hang appropriate work, to celebrate the aesthetic achievements of the youngsters.

Suggested spaces: front office, library, cafeteria, secretarial area in the office.

2. Maintain an ongoing bulletin board with appropriate student work.

3. Set up a movable art therapy booth in high traffic areas around the school. Provide an art therapy exhibit.

4. Develop an "Art Therapy Resource Kit" for pertinent school and program staff. Include your schedule and information about the field.

5. Share information about students at case conferences and other program meetings.

6. Have a group of students prepare a large artwork for the school (for example, a banner or group painting). Hang or display the piece and have a dedication ceremony. Invite school staff. Serve refreshments and honor the student achievement.

7. Arrange for an art therapy educational or artistic display in the community. Select such sites as the local library or hospital.

8. Send a press release to the media describing a unique art therapy project, and invite the reporters to the school to see the activity in action.

9. Provide staff development sessions to school groups. Also, meet with the principal and other school administrators as often as possible.

10. Provide an inservice on art therapy to the school PTA/PTSA (Parent-Teacher-Student Association group).

11. Write an article about your program for publication in a local community newspaper. If the article is printed, duplicate copies and distribute them to school staff.

12. Ask your school administrators if you can help them in any way, for example, by doing an assessment on a youngster in need. The youngster does not have to be in your program schedule. Show your administrators that you are interested in the general welfare of the school and students.

13. Conduct program special events such as art shows, field trips, artist of the week, chalk-ins, and other art therapy-type happenings.

14. Invite administrators to observe art therapy in action. Prepare a written "open invitation."

15. Maintain your art therapy space, materials, and equipment in an orderly and attractive way.

16. Always be on time for school and sessions.
17. Prepare an idea sheet of art/communication/feeling ideas for school personnel to use in the classroom or counseling sessions.
18. Plan a special event for a day's celebration or for a week-long celebration of "Art Therapy" activities.
19. Give out art therapy "coupons" to teachers, containing statements like "The bearer of this coupon can send students to Art Therapy for a 10-minute Art-Break."
20. Sponsor a "coffee in the faculty lounge" session with a "thank you" note to the staff for its interest and cooperation.
21. Set up a checkout bookshelf in the library with teacher and student books related to art therapy, feelings, etc.
22. Develop a parent bulletin—telling parents about your services and when you are available.
23. Schedule and show art therapy films for the staff, and counseling-type films for the children.
24. Sponsor art therapy-related activities during lunch hour.
25. Conduct a mini-inservice on stress management and relaxation through art for school staff.
26. Prepare an Art Therapy Goody Bag for each teacher. Enclose several activities that can be used with the students; include "scrap" art supplies.
27. Call the local media to help promote your creative projects.
28. Maintain good rapport with your school's art teacher. Seek suggestions and ideas for art-related activities, motivations, and art materials.
29. Encourage students to become fluent in a variety of expressive modes.
30. Utilize notebooks for sketches and thoughts.
31. Maintain individual student portfolios for assessing progress.
32. Allow teachers and administrators to experience art-counseling techniques. Through experience, they may gain some new understanding of themselves and may bring new depth to their work with the children.
33. Recommend books and other resources to teachers.
34. Be available for followup discussions and interactions with teachers.
35. Promote parent education groups—e.g., family art workshops.
36. Provide thank you notes to teachers who have done a good job in implementing tasks you have suggested.

37. See that all newsworthy events in your school and program are reported to local newspapers.
38. Encourage teachers, administrators, parents, and others to speak out for art therapy.
39. Maintain up-to-date information about what art therapists are thinking, writing, and saying. Keep aware of trends and ideas in the field.
40. Take advantage of opportunities to talk about the values of art therapy to persons and groups in the community—parents, business persons, school board members, clergy, community leaders, neighbors, and the general public.
41. Send notes to teachers and parents to inform them of their child's achievement.
42. Contribute articles to a local student services newsletter. Develop an ongoing "art therapy column." Suggested topics:

    a. Paraphrased articles, with reference citations from professional art therapy journals, that deal with emotionally disturbed children/adolescents
    b. Art therapy as a facilitator of behavioral change
    c. Art therapy for building self-esteem
    d. Group art therapy to improve social interaction
    e. Art therapy for an adolescent student
    f. Facilitating emotional goals through art therapy
    g. Working with a multidisciplinary team
    h. Problem-solving through art therapy
    i. An art therapy technique (one that is unique to art therapy that you have had success with)
    j. The interplay of cognitive and emotional development in art therapy
    k. Art therapy as an indicator of behavioral and emotional change
    l. Art therapy and improved body image

Be professional! Love yourself and what you do!

Summary of Steps to Follow in Carrying Out the Strategies

Decide on the target audience (PTA, parents, teachers, administrators, the general public). Decide where the funds will come from to prepare slide presentations, videos, posters, etc. Work with committee members to share responsibilities. Publicize the activities in the newspaper, on the radio, on TV. Follow up activities with reports to the newspapers, and with letters of appreciation for assistance.

PUBLIC RELATIONS AND THE MEDIA

A relationship with the news media—television, radio, and the newspapers—can result in opportunities to communicate many positive things that are happening with a program, and can educate your community about art therapy. It cannot only generate an ongoing interest in art therapy, but can prevent misinformation from spreading. It will not only assist in promoting the accomplishments of students and staff, but will contribute to the enhancement of a specialized professional means of dealing effectively with mental and emotional hangups that beset students and impede their ability to function at an optimum level in the classroom.

Making Contact Through Press Releases

Sending out a concise press release describing an activity is the first step to take in contacting the media. The information is intended to promote awareness. Include the date, time, and place, as well as the name and phone number of the art therapist/contact person. Indicate whether photo opportunities will be available.

Before preparing a press release, discuss your plans with key staff members. Remember, working with the media is viewed as a positive experience, not extra work! In discussing your ideas with staff, generate the excitement attached to media exposure.

Once a release has been developed, it should be mailed to the attention of appropriate media contact persons, for example, the education writer, the editor, the bureau chief of an agency. If the media are interested, they will usually telephone to arrange an appointment. If there has been no response after a press release has been sent, you may want to follow up with a telephone call to the appropriate contact person. The media are usually cooperative, and if they are interested in creating a story, they will visit the activity. If, however, they do not view your event as newsworthy, they will probably not respond.

A good press release highlights something that will draw the attention of the press. It details information in a clear and engaging manner— geared to persuade the press that your program activity is the most important thing happening in the news that day! A sample letter requesting media coverage and a sample press release are shown in Appendix K and Appendix L.

Subjects for Feature Stories

Generally, the use of art as a therapeutic tool is sufficient to warrant media attention. Sometimes, however, the media may be interested in special activities. A therapeutic theme and a special activity that did not fail to evoke media interest coincided in the presentation of students in the Dade County Public Schools working out emotional issues through drawing activities following their experience with Hurricane Andrew. Other occasions for interest might be community issues or holiday events. The focus is, of course, on how students cope with a particular problem, and on why the art therapy experience is valuable for them.

Other suggestions are:

- Student presentations
- Field trips
- Guest speakers
- Preparation of a unique art project
- An unusual experience in the local community
- Teachers participating in hands-on inservice
- A schoolwide project

Additional topics of interest may be:

- A particular student or staff member relating to a special individual experience, project, or event.
- The progress of a student in art therapy.
- The involvement of a staff member or the entire school staff in art therapy.
- The uniqueness of art therapy itself—how art therapy is assisting troubled youngsters to express their problems.
- Parent participation—workshops or other programs in which parents participate.
- An administrator or community leader who backs the art therapy program and who helps to support the services.
- What children's artwork means—explaining children's expression at various ages would be of special interest to parents to help them understand what their children are communicating.
- Conferences and seminars of local, statewide, or national interest.

How Art Therapists Should Prepare for Media Visits

There is frequently little lead time to prepare for media visits. Once a press release is sent, media personnel may want to visit right away. Art therapists must be prepared for a visit if releases have been sent. The following steps can be taken to ensure a positive visit:

1. Discuss the activity with appropriate staff members prior to the visit. Inform them of your plans.
2. Maintain a current list of students who have press/photo releases on file. Art therapists should oversee the completion of release forms related to participation in such art therapy projects as exhibits, press photos, and the use of artwork for professional educational purposes. Art therapists should ensure that students have releases on file and available during the visit with the press. Any youngsters who do not have a release and who cannot have a photo taken or their artwork viewed should not be included in an activity.
3. It is the art therapist's responsibility to make all arrangements for the day of the visit. When necessary, this includes providing information to appropriate staff members and parents. An effort should be made to help the visit go as smoothly as possible, without adding extra tasks for other personnel.
4. Highlights of a student's positive experiences in art therapy may be provided, and handouts on art therapy may be made available in the form of a "press packet." However, you must be discreet in sharing information about particular youngsters. Confidentiality must be maintained when relating stories about students.

POLITICAL INVOLVEMENT OF ART THERAPISTS

Political action is a part of public relations. It means finding a way to reach and influence policy makers whose decisions will affect art therapy. Sometimes individual art therapists can put across their personal ideas to policy makers, but it often takes the united effort of a group of art therapists, operating within the national, state, or local art therapy organization, to exert influence on the setters of policy.

An art therapist alone cannot easily reach a state governor or a U.S. Congressperson or have an impact on the state department of education or the state legislature, but an art therapy association, sometimes working closely with other related professional groups, can become a powerful force. Political action involves careful planning and a united effort in order to reach the policy makers and to help them recognize the values of art therapy, or to enlist their support of present programs and needed changes.

In this time of public concern over the cost and goals of all aspects of education, art therapists must unite to maintain control over their profession and its inclusion in educational settings.

The audiences to be reached by political action include the individuals or groups that make policies which affect art therapy at local, state, and national levels, and other sources that can be influential in the decision-making: local school boards, superintendents, and principals; local government officials such as mayors, council members, and judges; state legislators; directors and supervisors for subjects and programs in state departments of education; and members of Congress. Agencies and group organizations should also be included: PTA, Chamber of Commerce, arts and mental health councils, clergy, political leaders, business people, administrators, and other dignitaries.

Effective political action requires building close communication and rapport with all audiences in the local, state, and even national communities. It is a long and arduous process that needs consistent development, planning, and implementation.

Some suggestions for political action are:

- Make a list of all policy makers at the local and state levels who might affect art therapy. Whenever possible, get to know the individuals.
- Send the policy makers occasional art therapy publications.
- Send the policy makers letters that emphasize art therapy in the State.
- Ask the policy makers to speak at art therapy conferences. Publicize the speakers in the newspapers.
- Ask dignitaries to attend art therapy professional events as guests. Publicize their attendance.
- Find ways to publicly recognize those who support art therapy; present them with awards, certificates, or citations.
- Ask those who support art therapy to write statements on art therapy for journals and newsletters.
- Share publications.

• Develop close cooperation with and understanding of departments in colleges and universities. If they do not have art therapy training, help to inform and educate the departments on the meaning and value inherent in art therapy.

CONFIDENTIALITY AND RELEASE FORMS

In maintaining ethical responsibility toward clients and the therapeutic relationship, it is important for art therapists to be sensitive to the need to expose art products and background information only in ways approved by the American Art Therapy Association (AATA, Ethical Standards for Art Therapists, 1994).

Many programs for students with special needs provide general consent forms for participation in special school activities. When students are included in such activities, art therapists must ensure that special art therapy forms accompany the general school program forms that are used.

A. Confidentiality

1. Records
   Under no circumstances may a student be identified before the public by name, address, or other specific information that may breach the student's privacy. Identification may simply be by sex and age. IDEA (Individuals with Disabilities Education Act) provides confidentiality for every disabled child by declaring all records confidential. Distribution of records is based upon written consent by parents or guardians.
2. Artwork
   Under no circumstances may a student's art therapy products be displayed without written consent. Consent must be in the form of specific use of the product, date, place, and purpose of the exhibit. Any accompanying brochures with the exhibition of a student's art therapy products must also have written consent (Canon IV, Sections A and B, and Canon V, Sections A and B of the code of Ethical Responsibility of the American Art Therapy Association, September 1990).
3. Photographing Art

Written consent should be obtained to photograph student works of art for any purpose including:
(a) Public presentation at professional conferences
(b) Inservice presentations
(c) Research
(d) Exhibits
(e) Reproduction with accompanying articles to be submitted for publication to professional journals
(f) Videotapes
(g) Film

Sample Consent Forms 1, 2, and 3 appear in Appendix M.

B. Release Forms

Note: Individuals wishing to obtain consent from parents and schools for the use of student art therapy products must provide release forms that outline their intent, and give their agreement to abide by the rules. The specific use of the product, the date, the place, and the purpose must be specified before the signatures of the students' parents or legal guardians may be obtained. Release forms must be kept on file with the consent forms issued by the school.

Chapter 13

PROGRAM FUNDING STRATEGIES

The most difficult obstacle to overcome in the provision of art therapy services is often the procurement of funds. A basic budget for a program includes such expenditures as personnel costs for full-time or part-time services and, if available, for fringe benefits, as well as for art supplies. A more enhanced budget would include funding for training—money required for the hiring of consultants to give direction to art therapists and other interested personnel. Travel monies are needed to attend conferences and meetings, and funds must be provided for such professional resources as books and publications. The specific amounts budgeted for each of these areas depends upon individual programs and schools. Schools that can adopt an enhanced budget are obviously in a better position to carry out a comprehensive program.

Where will the monies come from? A variety of sources are available, but it may be up to individual art therapists to explore the possibilities for acquiring the funds. Sources include federal funding, locally generated monies, grants, and funds from business and industry. A combination of strategies may have to be employed to obtain sufficient resources to operate effectively.

Funds can be designated for art therapy through IDEA (Individuals with Disabilities Education Act)—the reauthorization act for Public Law 94-142 (The Education for All Handicapped Children Act)—as long as eligible candidates for treatment are identified and there is a qualified art therapist to provide the art therapy services. Public school districts receive monies for disabled children from the federal funds generated by this Public Law. If school districts choose, they can budget and pay for all of the expenses incurred for art therapists from this funding source. Usually, however, school districts do not consider art therapy a high priority in the funding chain, and every penny is accounted for elsewhere. Individual art therapists themselves may be the key to educating administrators to the benefits inherent in an art therapy approach, and they may also be best able to persuade the districts to budget for art therapy expenses.

Federal funds through IDEA are not available for youngsters who are not identified as disabled. However, there may be other federal monies available through other school programs or departments, such as alternative education programs, or remedial education programs, and through special diagnostic, evaluation, and research programs. School districts often receive federal assistance for a variety of youngsters, for example, those needing support services to receive the maximum benefits from education. Art therapy can aid such youngsters in reaching their maximum potential.

The grass roots approach to the funding of art therapy services and programs is through locally generated dollars. The sources are usually tax revenues, monies for individual districts allocated from the state department of education, or tuition monies if a private school organization is involved. It is up to the local school, district, or private school organization to make local budget funds available for art therapy.

Schools would have to view art therapy as a necessity before they would allocate the expenditures required. The Dade County Public Schools has recognized the need for art therapists since 1979, and has integrated them into the exceptional student education programs. The personnel costs for all of the full-time art therapists and the art supply budgets have both been paid for through local school monies.

Grants offer excellent possibilities for securing art therapy funding. Federal, state, and local grants are advertised in a variety of publications, such as The Foundation Directory, the Catalogue of Federal Domestic Assistance, and the Annual Register of Grant Support. These publications may be found in a public library. Grant-funded programs can cover all or part of art therapy expenses, depending on the amount of money involved. If grant monies are small, for example, $4,000, they can be used as seed money or to secure matching funds. Art therapy services can also be divided among several grant sources, for example, personnel costs from one grant source and supply money from another grant source.

Applications for grants are available from a variety of sources. State Arts Councils, usually based in a capital city, offer monies for direct services for special populations. A "Community Arts Development Grant" may be utilized to expand arts services in a community; for example, by providing "expressive arts counseling" to promote arts awareness in an at-risk middle school population, a population that may seldom be reached by the arts.

State Arts Councils provide Technical Assistance Grants that may be used for activities that do not involve direct student services, for example, the developing and administering of art therapy assessments and evaluations, or the providing of training programs for school staff.

State Arts Councils can assist in securing grants for "Artists in Residence programs." These activities are designed for direct work with special populations. Art therapy may well be best provided through this route.

Other sources for grants, besides State Arts Councils, may be found by contacting the National Endowment for the Arts (NEA), in Washington, D.C., and the Very Special Arts (VSA) Programs at both the state and federal levels.

Many private corporations and businesses are supporters of an array of services, activities, and special efforts designed to promote community involvement. Art therapists may want to contact the various offices of large and small companies and speak with personnel in charge of corporate grants. They are likely to be found in community relations, public relations, and corporate development departments designated to engage in outreach programming efforts and funding. Inquiring about types of programs, grants, and creative projects may be the start of developing art therapy services for special school populations.

Other businesses may also be approached to request funding donations for art supplies and materials that could be used expressly for an art therapy program.

The media, including TV and radio stations, may have opportunities such as an "Art That Heals" campaign, through which they can support an ongoing exhibit, and even services, for needy special populations.

Another vehicle for funding art therapy services and programs involves an opportunity for employment by a mental health or arts agency that may be able to contract for the provision of art therapy services to school districts. Individuals employed in this capacity are often able to expand services to include a school population.

It is important to note that a suggested strategy for obtaining funding for services and programs for a school population may involve the need to avoid clinical and medical terms when appealing to arts or education funders, and to utilize instead such terminology as "expressive arts counseling" or "communicating through art." These terms may be more meaningful than the term *art therapy* to those who provide the funding. The term *art therapy* is sometimes misunderstood or misinterpreted. If a proposal sounds overly oriented to mental health, it may be rejected on that basis (Malchiodi, 1987). The securing of funding for art therapy services and programs may also run into the tapping of funding for a population that has either been excluded from art services or underserved by art services. Donated funding, i.e., grants, is often provided to populations that are seldom served. It is important to keep this in mind as a strategy for obtaining funds when developing special projects for grants.

When all else fails, individuals may consider combining sources and strategies. Budgets among the sources can be shared. Local school-generated monies could fund personnel costs, and a grant could fund supplies; or 50 percent of an art therapist's time/costs could be funded from one source and the other 50 percent could be funded from another source; or 50 percent of an art therapist's time/costs could be funded from one school and the other 50 percent could be funded from a second school that the art therapist may serve. Time and costs do not have to be equal; they can be divided based on the availability of funds from specific areas, and based on the needs of individual programs.

Another option is for the art therapist to expand his/her role and carry out an additional responsibility that may meet a funding requirement of a particular source, or to be able to provide a service that a particular school needs assistance with. This strategy was employed in Dade County during the beginning years of the program. Emphasis was placed on the training of art teachers in techniques for use with disabled children. The art therapists allocated almost 50 percent of their time to providing a series of training programs for the art teachers. The results of this approach were twofold: The art education program could supply the strategies needed to assist the art teachers and their students, and the administrative concerns for providing teacher training were met, while funding was in place. Some critics of this approach termed it a prostitution of the art therapy service. It was not, however, a watering down of service; it was a way to emphasize additional roles that many qualified art therapists were capable of performing. Furthermore, it was evident that the goals of both the schools and the art therapists for this special student population were served. It was a "working example" of creative art therapy in action.

Developing Written Proposals

Information prepared in a proposal format will facilitate and expedite the review process that is needed to assess recommendations for new programs or for program improvement. Proposals should be no longer than five pages and should include:

- **Title and a 100-word Abstract:** Indicate potential value and impact of the project at local, state, and national levels.
- **Description:** Include the need for the project (rationale), goals and objectives, procedures, the calendar of events, strategies and activities, the method of evaluation and assessment, and the proposed final outcome.
- **Analysis of Project Impact:** Describe the potential impact of the project locally (value to the applicant and connection with his/her School Improvement Plan), the statewide value to schools, and the national value.
- **Budget:** Include a detailed, itemized project budget indicating the use of all funds (both cash and in-kind). Usually, funds may not be used for the purchase of equipment, T-shirts, salaries, bus rental, or indirect costs of administration. Funds may be used for guest artists, printing, postage, resources, materials, supplies, and other direct expenses. Indicate any supplementary funding sources (including cash match and in-kind contributions) that comprise a portion of the total project budget.
- **Timeline:** State your schedule for planning, development, implementation, and evaluation. Keep within expected deadlines.
- **Background of Applicant:** Include a summary of your professional background, experience in education, art therapy with school or school-related populations, and professional development as it relates to the proposed project. A resume may be included.
- **Community and Administrative Support:** Include at least two letters of support, preferably from school administrators such as principals or subject supervisors; parents; and college, university, or agency personnel.
- **Collaborating Individuals, Agencies, and Organizations:** List participating individuals, agencies, and organizations that will provide support for the proposed project.

To receive a favorable review of a proposal, adapt the language and style to correspond to the purpose of the potential funder.

Chapter 14

STANDARDS TO BE MET
IN SCHOOL ART THERAPY

The quality and level of support provided with art therapy services, as in other curriculum and service areas, differ greatly from one school to another and from one school district to another. In some communities, where art therapy is already a sustained tradition, and where it has been incorporated into established school policies, quality standards may exist. Administrative improvements can be suggested and dealt with. In other communities, where art therapy programs are struggling and are not yet developed, quality standards are useful as guidelines, but should not be discouragingly remote from current possibilities.

The American Art Therapy Association has been drafting comprehensive standards for school art therapy services. When the standards are available, they will assist individuals and groups in providing the programs and services, and will be deemed the approved guidelines to follow in implementing school programs. The hope is that they will help to validate and advance the use of art therapy.

The following domains relate to the quality standards for schools, and provide a measure on which good school art therapy should depend (adapted from the draft of School Art Therapy Standards of Practice of the American Art Therapy Association, 1994).

I. Policy
The state and district should have written educational goals that include art therapy. Presentations on art therapy should be part of all reports to the school board, state department of education, and individual schools.

II. Program Intent
A districtwide director, supervisor, coordinator, or chairperson should be on hand to lead art therapy. Art therapy should be conducted by professionals credentialed as registered art therapists

(A.T.R.) and Board Certified (B.C.). The focus of art therapy should be on assisting youngsters to work through emotional problems, not on getting them to appreciate art for art's sake. To be effective, art therapy must be appropriately scheduled, with adequate time allocated for necessary treatment. It should not be sandwiched in between other school activities and classes, leaving inadequate time to provide meaningful treatment services.

III. **Treatment Intent**

Art therapy can provide access to understanding a youngster's development both in the cognitive and emotional categories. Written guidelines and procedures that can be referred to and adhered to should undergird the "casualty treatment" that art therapy undertakes to administer. A valid and reliable assessment tool should be utilized as a reporting procedure to provide measures of a student's progress and development. Specific goals should be written, and an art therapy treatment plan implemented for each student served. Feedback on student progress should be reported to school staff and parents. Art therapy should be considered a real therapy in its own right, as important as such other school mental health interventions as school psychology and counseling. Art therapy should be related to the overall school program so it can contribute its own unique insights into developing goals and objectives for successful student educational plans. It can contribute meaningful information to the school treatment team that would not be available elsewhere. The artwork and sessions represent the concept of problem recognition/problem solution. The students complete activities that help them to express feelings, thoughts, imagination, and creative perceptions. The art therapists guide them to process their feelings and thoughts in conjunction with their artwork, and to verbalize them. Proper art therapy schedules must be in effect so that the art therapists can deal with caseloads of not more than 20 to 25 students a week, scheduled in small groups and individual settings. Confidentiality must be maintained to protect the identity of the students served.

IV. **Art Therapy Process**

When materials and concepts are introduced, guidance must be provided. Art therapists must have an understanding of the student artwork and behavior and must use intervention skills appropriately. Art therapists should demonstrate a therapeutic alliance with the students. Art therapists should relate to the students with respect. Art therapists should display concerned and caring attitudes toward the students. Art therapists should help the students to feel accepted even when they proscribe certain student behaviors. The students must receive individual attention. The students must be encouraged to explore their thoughts and feelings. The students must be led to use appropriate behavior. The students must be led to involve themselves in the cooperative care of materials and in the cleanup. The art therapists should then engage in evaluation and closure.

V. Documentation

The art therapists must follow professional record-keeping procedures. A variety of reports must be made: e.g., daily reports on student sessions; art products; art therapy assessments; goal, objective, and treatment plans; student progress reports. Findings must be reported to appropriate school treatment team members and parents. Clerical support should be provided to the art therapists for the preparation of the documentation records. The art therapists should have access to computers to insure efficiency of operation in all of the record-keeping procedures. Locked storage must be available for the retention of the art therapy records.

VI. Physical Conditions and Equipment, Materials, and Supplies

There must be an adequate appropriation of funds in the school system budget for each art therapist. There should be an appropriate amount of space to conduct art therapy privately. The environment, arranged through space, furnishings, equipment, materials, organization, and accessibility, must be compatible. The necessary art supplies must be available so the art therapist can implement a comprehensive art therapy program fully. General office supplies, as well as supplies for painting, drawing, collage, printmaking, sculpture, photography, and crafts must be accessible. Proper equipment to carry out an effective program includes a ceramic wheel, a kiln, water, safe and adequate electricity, and a paper cutter. The necessary expendable materials must be provided for every student; e.g., paint, paper, clay, brushes. Computers should be available for the new applications of computer art.

VII. Professional Development

A regularly scheduled program of professional inservice workshops and seminars on art therapy and related topics is essential. Art therapists should receive release time to attend conferences and professional events. Art therapists should be involved in assessing the art therapy programs/ services in order to meet the demands of change. Art therapists should have an opportunity to make presentations on their programs, to discuss the values of art therapy, and to exhibit appropriate student artwork. Above all, art therapists should be used as local resources for the purpose of conducting staff development workshops for all other personnel in the school district and for the community.

Chapter 15

RESEARCH NEEDS

The clinical use of art therapy is well established. Clinical art therapy is widely accepted both in public and in private psycho-educational settings, and it enjoys increasing recognition and respect. Art therapy in schools, however, has not yet taken root. The time for controlled research on the application of art therapy in school settings is now. However, since considerable skepticism exists regarding the efficacy of psychotherapy in general, a firm stand—negative or positive—on the merits of school art therapy cannot be taken until many new results of application and feedback have been studied and quantified. It will take time to establish relevant outcome criteria, and to find answers to a number of questions, among them: Across what dimension should change be assessed? What is the appropriate magnitude for any given child?

Change in attitude or behavior or capability can be externally defined with the help of parents, teachers, and other agents in a position to observe. Change can also be defined through readiness for success in mainstream education or through return to a regular public school program. It can be further defined through a child's self-reports or through analysis of a child's artwork and comments.

What is needed initially is a foundation for thought. The publication of accounts on the relative effectiveness of art therapy application to students in the schools, following controlled investigation and the use of a variety of methodologies by the schools, could serve as a base. Research would provide objective and empirical verification of the principles underlying art therapy and of selected case outcomes. Forums based on the research could spur individual scientific research workers and art therapists to engage in a concerted effort to have art therapy included in school programs for all children.

By comparing conclusions and linking them to information arrived at in clinical settings, additional knowledge could be gained. Similarities and differences emerging from the results of the work carried on with clinical and school populations could make refined opinions possible.

Other comparisons could be made through anecdotal accounts and by means of chronicled situations that reflect accurate historical records of events.

Cumulative documentation will give rise to firm negative and positive positions on the subject, and will not fail to bring up the many questions that people will ponder. The end result should be movement—hopefully, movement toward the benign introduction of school art therapy for all children who need it—in all public schools.

Chapter 16

THE CHALLENGE AHEAD

We are constantly reminded that we must prepare our students for the twenty-first century. This challenge for the future, while good, has revealed numerous cracks in the road. Scores of children are physically and mentally unhealthy, and their environment is not equipped to bring out the best in them. An increasing number of them are living in poverty, and suffering from the deterioration of family and neighborhood ties. The dearth of essential services needed to create change in their lives is leading to a critical situation. If we are to be effective in fulfilling our hopes for the twenty-first century, we must deal with the cracks in the road now.

Art therapy can work quietly and steadily to improve the fit between children and education, and between children and their home and neighborhood environments. Art therapy is equipped to turn lives around by inducing salutary changes in attitude, which can, in turn, foster self-understanding and the effort to achieve. Art therapists can bring about the desire in students to self-identify and to concentrate on finding out what they like, what they do best, what they want out of life, and what paths to take to acquire personal happiness. Art therapists can concurrently instill the idea that satisfaction results from performing services for others. In substance, art therapists can inject the values of community and trust, responsibility and reliability, friendship and loyalty, learning and training, and worthiness as opposed to worthlessness in students. But considerable talent, energy, good will, and dollars will have to be expended, and treatment will have to become an integral part of instruction in every school.

The American Art Therapy Association (AATA) is becoming a strong force in encouraging state and national legislation on a wide range of social and educational issues; in advocating and structuring guidelines for graduate level training; in implementing standards for practice, and approval procedures for educational training programs; in developing national certification standards for the practice of professional art therapy;

in creating committees and task forces to promote education, ethics, and professional practice; in advocating governmental involvement in improving the conditions of life; and in planning for the future. Its actions and its support concepts have given art therapists a unique identity among the helping professions—an identity that signifies ability and readiness to repair and redirect the acting-out behaviors of students that have been triggered by broken emotions and that have consistently misdirected their energies.

It is risky to predict the future, but school art therapists who are in the business of helping others to prepare for the future must be ready to meet the challenges of a changing world. Projections for future school art therapists must take into account such weighty factors as philosophical and training concerns, programmatic issues, technological advances, an emerging global economy, and an altered variety of students and schools.

Reconceptualization of school art therapy as a field and of the other domains that relate to mental health must take place. We must maintain "quality in training" (Levick, 1978, 1989, 1994). We must redefine our training standards, learn a common language, and require the accountability of our members (Levick, 1994). Training art therapists to satisfy the needs of students and the demands of schools is a major issue. Training programs must establish proven criteria. Consistency in subject matter and procedure must be initiated. Courses and supervised clinic hours must be arranged to meet the requirements set forth by the American Art Therapy Association Education and Training Board.

Art therapy reflects a relationship between art and therapy. The relationship is a valid one, but our operations have straddled different approaches and philosophies of practice, which have interfered with harmonious results.

I discovered the problem of inconsistency in training in the early 1980s as the Dade County Public Schools Art Therapy Program began to grow. When additional art therapists were employed, our job became harder because we did not speak a common language. All of the art therapists on the staff came from different training and orientation programs. We were supposed to be a unified group, responding interchangeably to the demands of a large urban school system, but we were actually fragmented. In a case conference, we could display drawings on a board and report on a student's developmental milestones and the associations made as a by-product of the artwork. But we could not agree on clinical impressions, the possible symbolic meaning of the artwork, and the goals of the treatment. There was no common theoretical construct. Ultimately, we collaborated on a project with Dr. Levick and developed an art therapy assessment instrument, the Levick Emotional and Cognitive Art Therapy Assessment (Levick et al., 1989), which gave the group an opportunity to evaluate youngsters with one common instrument. By using the assessment as a planning tool for treatment, we were able to employ equivalent terminology when talking about the students and their problems. The assessment instrument paved the way for communication.

As we look to the twenty-first century, we know we must have training practices and approaches that are harmonious. Art therapists must pursue therapeutic ends. They are concerned with health, specifically cognitive and emotional health. Art teachers and professional artists, on the other hand, must concern themselves with academic, educational, and cultural aims. Art teachers and professional artists should teach technique and media skills. Their role is to improve the art products. Art therapists should not be doing the job of the art teacher or of the professional artist. Art therapists are needed to help sick individuals make contact with the practical material world. As health professionals, art therapists need to have a symbolic understanding of artwork and developmental issues if they are to succeed in their efforts to help individual students make connections that will resolve their conflicts, but art therapists should not concern themselves with the perfecting of the artistic qualities that are an intrinsic part of the products produced.

Leading students to produce artwork is not an end in itself, although it might be a cathartic experience for some. Art therapists must concentrate on helping their patients make the connections. They must focus on inducing some type of healing. This approach to art must involve special training (Levick, 1978, 1989, 1994).

A combined approach, demonstrated by the Dade County Public Schools Pilot Art Education Therapy Program in 1979, is well-suited to the task of dealing with the comprehensive needs of all children; it utilizes both concepts—the academic concept and the health concept. The pilot program, however, demonstrated that no one had been taking care of the emotional needs of the students involved—they needed psychotherapy. The postpilot years concentrated on the art therapy principles and practices called for.

I believe the preparation for understanding and applying the required "basics" of art therapy should be routine within every type of art therapy training program, and for every individual who wishes to practice art therapy, and that one genotype or species of art therapist should be trained both for art therapy in the schools and for art therapy in general. In-depth specialization should build on the "basics."

Good character is requisite for art therapists. They must be willing to grow, and willing to resolve their own conflicts, because they need to exercise high personal principles and standards that they adopt as behavioral habits to exert an untainted influence on the conduct of their students.

Teachers, counselors, school psychologists, and school social workers are experts schools hire to take care of nondisabled children, children with disabling conditions, and children with temporary social/emotional problems and learning deficits, but each category of expert performs discrete functions. To complete the team, there should be one expert who can bridge the gaps between all the other experts. The art therapist should be trained to perform this overlapping role.

Psychotherapy as a basis for the work of all art therapists must be taught and practiced. We cannot help children in schools and patients in clinical settings by having them just make art. We have to know how to help them explore the art they have produced and how to help them resolve their conflicts.

We cannot support individuals operating in art therapy environments who profess ideas revolving around the "magical," the "spiritual," or the "mystical" when interpreting a patient's artwork. They distort the identity of serious art therapists and confuse colleagues in other disciplines of mental health and education with their assumptions—their allusions to the occult tend to cast suspicion on our professional integrity (Levick, 1994). As art therapists, we must relate only to conditions and events that are recognizable in the functional world we inhabit.

We must consider who the students of the future will be and for what reasons they will seek assistance from school art therapists. If the present fragmenting trends in this country's families and culture are any indication, the students of the next century will be fighting the debasement of a variety of noble personal instincts and ideals and will need an array of special services to counter their downhill learning curve as well as their failure to utilize emotional strength, good morals, and wise judgment.

In serving the students of tomorrow, school art therapists will have to be prepared to address developmental needs, to prevent learning difficulties, and to recognize and remedy existing conditions that impair healthy emotional and cognitive growth, physical development, and behavior. All students of tomorrow will require instruction that helps them to develop skills, to acquire information, and to attain knowledge that can lead to appropriate decisions about relationships, educational goals, and aspirations—they will also need to be prepared to change their goals, to make adjustments, and to prevent major problems from blocking their progress. Students with special needs will require special assistance. To get through the school day and to access education, and, ultimately, life, appropriately, such students will need the concentrated, extended help of art therapists.

The changing American family structure has created new norms. Divorce, remarriage, cohabitation, dual careers, and blended families make up the array of current family structures. Each family, with its own set of beliefs, contributes in unique ways to the culture and values that each student brings to school. Therefore, each student's family lays the groundwork for the educational success or lack of success of the student.

Teenage pregnancy, sexually transmitted diseases, and a host of contingency problems of devastating proportions continue despite the availability of birth control and contraceptive education. Technological change, substance abuse, sexual activity, violence, disease, poverty, cultural and racial diversity, and many other conditions will continue to concern students, parents, and teachers, and school art therapists will need to be prepared to identify and treat the many problems that will arise, as well as to help prevent the problems from occurring in the first place.

The changing family structure is not the only concern—the social ills of society, e.g., drugs, are mounting. Although they continue to be countered, few victories and too many losses are evident. Babies who are born of drug abusing parents are entering our schools daily. Schools and art therapists face a major challenge in designing programs and services for such youngsters, who may be too infected by their addictions ever to realize their academic and emotional potential.

Unless violence is curtailed, it will be a phenomenon that will have significant impact on future schools and students. Physical, sexual, and psychological child abuse today proves that society has not yet properly protected the children. Added to the brutal violation of children's rights by some parents and adults is the use of force by a growing number of students as a means of addressing peer conflicts. Fights, homicides, and suicides are rampant within youth peer culture. Helping children of tomorrow to handle hostilities in appropriate ways while maintaining an acceptable level of assertiveness to protect their interests and enhance their welfare will be a necessary aspect of school life. Art therapists can take a leadership role in the effort both to stamp out crime and to divert student interests away from the attitudes that make them prone to involvement in lives of crime.

A sample of school art therapy job specifications that can serve now and in the future is shown in Appendix N.

As old issues are resolved, new issues will emerge to take their place. While the process of human development is expected to remain unchanged, the impact of a changing world on human development will remarkably alter aspects of the developmental process.

In the early 1900s, Alfred Adler, through his theory of individual psychology, concluded "that mental health can be measured in terms of one's social interest, and the willingness to participate in the give and take of life," and he felt that one should cooperate with others and be concerned about their welfare (Dinkmeyer, Dinkmeyer, and Sperry, 1987, p. 64). A similar concept of individualization is a theme for the twenty-first century predicted by Naisbitt and Aburdene (1990). The first principle, which these authors call "the triumph of the individual," is a belief in personal responsibility. The embracement of individual worth and responsibility is complemented by a spirit of togetherness and community, two other qualities that should be nurtured by school environments. Recognition of individual worth, combined with responsibility for personal behavior, suggests that individuals must come together and contribute to the betterment of all humankind. We cannot hope to flourish in the future if communities are composed of individuals who behave like strangers to one another and who are bent on harm.

Art therapists can contribute to a brighter future by helping students to improve their emotional and mental attitudes. Future school art therapists should be prepared to maintain comprehensive services to meet the needs of a wide range of students. We have to identify and resolve student problems if we wish to be in control of law and order in our lifetime. Helping students to establish healthy relationships and to choose responsible behaviors will be the most important role of the future.

We can accomplish the goal through the restructuring of student services in our schools. This is not a pipe dream. It is real! Student services, through art therapy, can be the medium for empowering change and improvement in student attitude, effort, character, and behavior.

My work in the Dade County Public Schools has taught me that dreams can have substance and can come true. I have learned that dreams are conceivable . . . then believable . . . then achievable. But one must be careful between believable and achievable because in between them is the possibility of encountering deceivable. I want to express a word of caution here. No amount of enthusiasm for an idea can shut out a dream stealer who says something cannot be done. We have to believe, if something is good, that it can indeed be done! And we have to pursue it until we achieve success!

Personal dedication helped me to prove that my dream was believable . . . and then achievable. My idea that art therapy will be an integral part of the education vision for the twenty-first century is believable, and can prove to be achievable.

The challenge ahead is to reinforce the efforts of individuals to reform our institutions, to prevent what is good from falling into disuse or disrepair, and to restore our faith in ourselves and others. We can and must change for the better; we can and must believe that we wish to change; and we can and must engage our talents, our energies, and our dollars to insure that there will be progress in change. Our creative use of art therapy to effect change can help our students to know who they are and what they are capable of. This action on our part cannot fail to teach them, more than anything else, what this nation is all about.

APPENDICES

APPENDIX A. SAMPLE REGULATIONS AND PROCEDURES FOR THE IEP (INDIVIDUALIZED EDUCATION PLAN)

Regulations and Procedures for the Individualized Education Plan

Copies of IDEA (Individuals with Disabilities Education Act) are free and can be obtained by writing your congressman. It is helpful to request copies of state regulations from State Boards of Education, since each state differs a little in the way it carries out the procedures governing the implementation of IDEA, and each individual school system establishes its own guidelines for implementing the law following state and federal guidelines. Art therapists should also contact their local school systems for guidelines in order to understand how to proceed in promoting an art therapy program in their local school system.

Under IDEA, the eligibility process and development of the IEP are the legal basis for including art therapy in special education programs. The IEP is designed to ensure that the assessed individual needs of a student are provided for. All related services are documented on the IEP. What follows in Part I is an abridged outline of the eligibility process. Part II details the inclusion of art therapy services in this process.*

Part I

ELIGIBILITY

1. Student Rights
   a. Under IDEA, eligible students are entitled to an individualized education program and related services that would benefit the children in their education.
2. Special Education Services
   a. The child must be 0–21 and identified as disabled.
3. Request for Special Education and Related Services
   a. Parental request
   b. Faculty request
      (1) Principal, teacher, school psychologist, other related service providers
4. Screening Process
   (The screening process allows for the identification of those students who need special education and related services)
   a. Referral
      (1) Student is referred to the screening committee, which reviews the referral and determines the need for evaluations and test procedures.

---

    b. Notification
        (1) Parental permission is required for evaluations to be conducted.
    c. Evaluation Procedure
        (1) Assessment of eligibility for special education and possible related
            services
            a. educational
            b. medical
            c. psychological
            d. socio-cultural
            e. developmental (pre-school)
            f. visual/hearing/speech/language (if applicable)
    d. Review
        (1) The screening committee reviews the results of all documented evalua-
            tions—the results are used later in developing the student's individual-
            ized education plan.
    e. Student Entitlements
        (1) Tests and evaluations should be nondiscriminatory and may be pro-
            vided by school personnel or by privately contracted individuals.
        (2) Testing and evaluating must be given by someone who has the proper
            training.
        (3) Tests cannot be given if they are inappropriate, and all screening
            methods given shall be appropriate regarding the developmental,
            educational, and functional levels of the student.
        (4) All test and evaluation results and all records are confidential and
            cannot be distributed without written permission from the parents.
5. Eligibility Meetings
    a. They serve to determine the eligibility of students for placement or contin-
        ued placement in the special education program.
6. Program Development
    a. Individualized Education Program (IEP)
        (1) Developed after eligibility for special education and related services
            has been decided.
        (2) Based on findings of the screening committee and eligibility meetings.
        (3) IEP addendums are provided for additions or revisions in the educa-
            tional program and/or related services after IEP has been developed
            (and before annual program review).
    b. IEP Content
        (1) Child's current level of performance
            (a) academic skills (test scores, etc.)
            (b) communication skills
            (c) social/emotional adaptation and behavior
            (d) pre-vocational/vocational skills
            (e) psychomotor skills/physical education (gross motor)
            (f) self-help skills
        (2) Annual goals and short term objectives

      (3) Special education and related services to be provided

      (4) Commencement date and anticipated duration of services (dates for initiating and terminating services)

      (5) Length of individual or group sessions (state length of session and number of sessions provided per week)

      (6) Description of service provider

      (7) Appropriate objective criteria, evaluation procedures, and schedules for determining (at least on an annual basis) whether short-term objectives have been achieved.

7. Program Implementation
   a. Based on IEP
8. Program Review
   a. Annual review of progress (or other scheduled date)
   b. Documentation of review in a narrative report
9. Annual IEP Meeting
   a. Members present
      (1) Representative of school (other than child's teacher) qualified to provide or supervise the provision of special education
      (2) The child's teacher
      (3) One or both parents or legal guardian or parent surrogate
      (4) Others, such as specialists in the child's condition and related service providers
   b. Purpose
      (1) Review IEP and placement
      (2) Revise IEP if necessary
         (a) deletion or addition of related services
         (b) deletion, revision, or addition of goals or objectives

Part II

DIRECT ART THERAPY SERVICES

1. Student Rights
   a. Art therapy is specified as a related service.
2. Special Education Services
   a. Art therapy can be provided to eligible students as a related service in order to enable the students to benefit from special education.
3. Request for Special Education and Related Services
   a. Parents can request an art therapy evaluation to determine the suitability of this related service for their child.
      (1) Initial request for special education and related services including art therapy.
      (2) Subsequent request after determined eligible and placed in special education program.

  b. Faculty Request
    (1) Principal, teacher, school psychologist, or other related service provider can request an art therapy evaluation for a student.
    (2) Art therapists can provide a list of characteristics for potential art therapy candidates to multi-disciplinary staff members who serve as referral sources.
4. Screening Process
  (For art therapy as a related service to special education)
  a. Referral
    (1) The school art therapist may implement a diagnostic art therapy assessment, or the parent may seek out a private art therapist for a private evaluation.
  b. Notification
    (1) The parent should be notified and should give consent to have the child screened by the staff art therapist.
  c. Evaluation Procedure
    (1) A diagnostic art therapy assessment may be administered at this time, when a request has been documented on a referral form; or at a later point in time, after psychological testing, a referral for an assessment may be forwarded by the school psychologist to determine eligibility for art therapy as a related service.
  d. Review
    (1) The art therapy assessment is reviewed and documented.
  e. Student Entitlements
    (1) The screening method used in the diagnostic art therapy procedure must be nondiscriminatory and may be provided by the school art therapist or by a privately contracted art therapist.
    (2) The art therapist should hold a master's degree in art therapy or equivalent.
    (3) The art therapy evaluation procedure shall be appropriate regarding the developmental, educational, and functional levels of the student.
    (4) All art therapy evaluation results and all records are confidential and cannot be distributed without written permission from the parents.
        (a) For the art therapist this includes exhibiting the student's works of art, presenting slides identified by name, or including the student's face, etc. (AATA's Code of Ethical Responsibility, September, 1990 also makes reference to confidentiality.)
        (b) The art therapist can design a release form to use for requisitioning parental permission for exhibiting student's works of art, etc.
5. Eligibility Meetings
  a. The eligibility of the student for special education is determined.
    (1) This determination may include art therapy services, or referral for art therapy services may occur after placement in the special education program.
6. Program Development
  a. Individualized Education Program (IEP)

(1) The IEP is developed based on the student's needs, not based on the availability of services.

    (a) Art therapy should be included on the IEP based on need, whether or not an art therapist is employed at the student's particular school.

    (b) Art therapy is written into the IEP based on the information disclosed in the documented diagnostic assessment.

  b. Content

    (1) Student's current level of functioning

    (2) Statement of annual art therapy goal and short-term art therapy objectives

    (3) Statement of art therapy as a related service

    (4) Commencement date and anticipated duration of art therapy services

    (5) Length of individual and/or group sessions

    (6) Description of service provider (art therapist)

7. Program Implementation

  a. The art therapist implements the treatment plan based on the IEP.

  b. The art therapist selects the methods, materials, and environmental structure necessary to accomplish the objectives.

  c. The art therapist monitors and modifies the treatment plan in order to achieve the objectives.

8. Program Review

  a. Annual review of progress (or other scheduled date)

  b. Documentation of review in an art therapy narrative report

    (1) Review of progress attained

      (a) Detailing progress and strategies in the course of treatment.

    (2) Recommendations

      (a) Continuation or termination of art therapy services

      (b) Addition, deletion, revision of art therapy objectives

9. Annual IEP Meeting

  a. Members present

    (1) An art therapist may be present at this meeting in order to orally discuss the student's progress, eligibility, or continued eligibility for art therapy services, and to answer any questions regarding the individualized art therapy program.

    (2) The presence of an art therapist may be beneficial if art therapy is being proposed as an additional service to be added to the IEP—at this time an oral presentation can be invaluable in persuading the committee that this service is necessary for the particular child.

APPENDIX B. SAMPLE PARENTAL CONSENT FORM FOR AN ART THERAPY ASSESSMENT

PARENTAL CONSENT FOR AN ART THERAPY ASSESSMENT

Date _____

_____ School _____
_____ Contact Person: _____
_____ Address: _____
_____ Telephone Numbers: _____

Dear _____:

Based upon a recommendation by _____, we are seeking
                              (Title of Professional)
your permission to provide your child, _____, with an art therapy
                                        (Child's Name)
assessment to help plan an educational program and services that best meet his/her needs.
School personnel have carefully reviewed your child's educational records and have
agreed that an assessment would help to determine the child's needs.

A specialist in school art therapy will administer the following instrument:

_____.

Indicate your choice below:

☐   **YOU HAVE MY PERMISSION** to conduct the assessment described.

☐   **I DO NOT GIVE** my permission for an assessment.

☐   **A CONFERENCE IS REQUESTED** to discuss the proposed assessment before I
     grant permission.

_____   _____
(Child's Name)   (Date of Birth)

_____   _____
(Parent's Signature)   (Date)

APPENDIX C. SAMPLE ASSESSMENT
ART THERAPY PROGRAM
ASSESSMENT REPORT

NOTE: Correct name withheld to protect the identity of the subject.

STUDENT NAME: __John Franklin__   DATE OF BIRTH: <u>January 29, 1982</u>

DATE(S) OF ASSESSMENT: <u>9/24/91 & 10/1/91</u>   ART THERAPIST: <u>Janet Bush, A.T.R.</u>

SCHOOL: __Children's Development Center__

Reason for Assessment

Further information was needed to assess functioning and to determine possible goals and objectives for art therapy treatment.

Highlights of Clinical History

John was the product of an uncomplicated pregnancy and delivery at term with subsequently normal development milestones. He experienced major traumas when his parents were divorced, when his father was shot and died, and when his mother got sick and died. John was abused prior to his mother's death. He was subsequently cared for by his grandmother, but most recently, has been in the custody of a maternal aunt and uncle. There were four children in John's original family. John currently lives with one sibling, while the other two siblings live with an aunt in Miami. One brother is retarded. John has no past medical history of risk factors. School history reflects uncontrollable outbursts of violent behavior, including destruction of school furniture and equipment.

Clinical Observation

John was shy and cooperative. He approached the drawing tasks with ease. When asked to respond verbally, he was quite hesitant, and provided little information. He frequently smiled when questions were asked of him.

Procedure

The Levick Emotional and Cognitive Art Therapy Assessment (LECATA) was administered. In a time period of approximately 60 minutes, the student was to complete six drawing tasks and title each one: a drawing of anything and a story about the drawing; a self-portrait; a scribble using one color; a picture created from the scribble; a place; and his family. The materials used were white 12″ × 18″ paper; a variety of colored oil pastel crayons; and a lead pencil with an eraser, which was available on request. This therapist observed the student at work during the assessment, and invited comments on the artwork.

Assessment Results

The criteria for scoring The LECATA are based on *The Correlation of Developmental Lines of Cognitive, Artistic, Psychosexual Sequences and Defense Mechanisms of The Ego Appropriate for Those Periods of Development* (Levick, 1983) and *Criteria for Identifying Defenses Manifested in Graphic Productions* (Levick, 1983). Based on the artistic representations, John's average cognitive score reflects development at age 6.4 years; his average emotional score reflects development at age 6.4 years. The combined average score reflects developmental functioning at the age of 6.4 years.

The low cognitive and emotional scores that John received in relation to his chronological age suggests that he may be experiencing a developmental delay that may be related to emotional difficulties. Psychological testing, including testing for learning disabilities and personality projectives, may more clearly define John's problem areas.

Overall, John's drawings manifest themes of loneliness and separation. The emotional defenses utilized are incorporation, denial, isolation, isolation of affect, regression, and imitation. These are low-level defenses in comparison with John's chronological age group, suggesting his needs to defend himself against unresolved issues of separation anxiety, fear of loss of control, and identification issues. John's traumatic early childhood has no doubt contributed to his unresolved emotional development issues. This is a youngster in need of much environmental support to assist him in working through his anger and the losses he has experienced.

In Task One, a picture of anything, John has created a colorful bird's-eye view of the world (Figure 21). He did not provide a detailed story, as would a youngster in his chronological age group, but he did provide the following description: "Someone is rushing to get off the Earth and go to Pluto; the title is "The Planet Earth." In this first picture task, John may be showing a habitual way of responding—he has portrayed a theme of separation—perhaps he does not feel grounded and connected to his environment. Cognitively, the drawing shows his strength of abstraction in perceiving the Earth from a distance. Shapes have been combined to make balanced forms, there is spatial organization, symbols and forms are encapsulated within other forms, and there is isolation seen in the object drawn singly on the page and separated from an environment.

In Task Two, a drawing of self, John used pencil to create a large figure of himself (Figure 22). He obtained a small mirror that was in the room and used it to look at himself as he drew. No color was applied in this drawing. There are rectangular shapes below the neck and the V-designs on John's shirt. He had great difficulty drawing the neck, the facial features, and lower body, and applied multiple erasures. Cognitively, this drawing shows a well-defined figure, but one that is lacking in detail and proportion. The drawing does show gender differentiation, which is an age-appropriate feature. In this task, we can view John's perception of himself. With wide, outstretched arms, he is presented as a vulnerable and fragmented self, almost compartmentalized. The figure lacks a sense of "wholeness."

In Tasks Three and Four, a scribble and a drawing from the scribble, John eagerly produced a scribble and depicted a darkened image of a tornado (Figure 23). This may manifest his turbulent and out-of-control feelings. He commented that he never

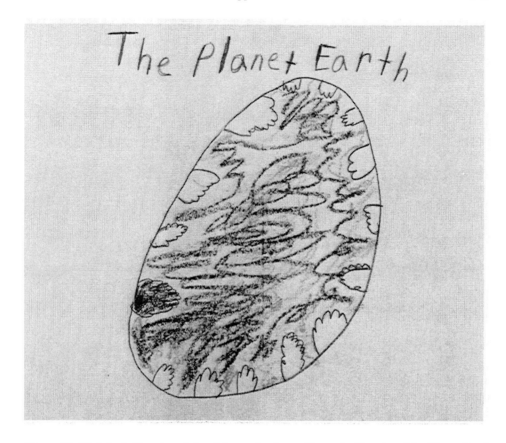

Figure 21. Task 1-A Drawing of Anything and a Story About the Drawing: The Planet Earth (John Franklin).

experienced a real tornado, but saw one on television, at which time he changed the television channel to watch cartoons. He had not liked what he had seen, and John's troubled tornado may represent another aspect of his troubled self and the world as he perceives it—isolated, destructive, and frightening. Turning the channel to watch cartoons may be an indication of his need to escape his unpleasant circumstances.

In Task Five, a place of importance, John created what he called, "A Picture Museum" (Figure 24). He showed the front of an elevator and described his scene as "a special place with a guard in a big building." John said that he had never been to a place like the one he drew, although he chose it as a place of importance. Cognitively, John has combined shapes to make balanced forms, yet the object is not readily identifiable—it appears more like doors that are tied and unable to be accessed.

This is an unusual response to the directive "Draw a Place of Importance," inasmuch as he had selected subject matter with which he said he had no familiarity. Perhaps John's image is representative of another place of importance, one which he

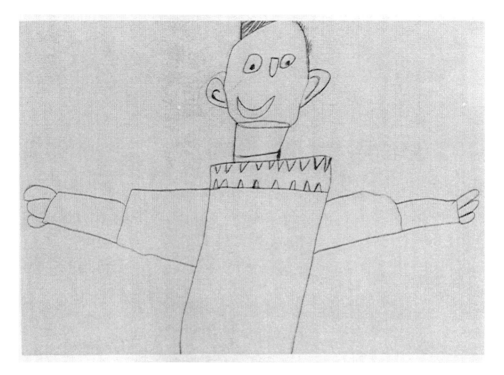

Figure 22. Task 2–Self-Portrait (John Franklin).

did not verbally or consciously identify, or perhaps it represents a wish to actually experience an art museum, or perhaps there is emotional significance in the bound doors, symbolically expressing accessibility to John's inner self.

In Task Six (Figure 25), his family, John experienced a great deal of anxiety—he started over several times and distracted himself by playing with some items that were on the table. From left to right, John drew his present family—Tania, an older sister; mom (his aunt); older brother, Gary; younger sisters, Sandy and Shanah; Cousin Morris; himself; and older brother, Martin. At the bottom of the page he drew his one-year-old nephew, who is depicted as crawling. The figures are not grounded, nor is there an environment. There is also a lack of interplay amongst the figures. These features may be indicative of a lack of interrelatedness within the home. Some of the figures are portrayed as sticks; others are full-bodied and clothed. It is difficult to ascertain gender differentiation. John's anxious behavior and conflicted drawing style indicate emotional unrest in his relationship with the family. John appears to be manifesting considerable depression, anxiety, and regression.

This is a youngster in need of opportunities to process the traumatic losses in his life: He needs conditions that permit him to mourn his losses and to learn how to assert anger in healthy and productive ways. The main finding that an observer might make from this series of tasks is that John shows feelings of isolation from people and from elements in the environment. Features that reflect this conclusion are portrayed in all

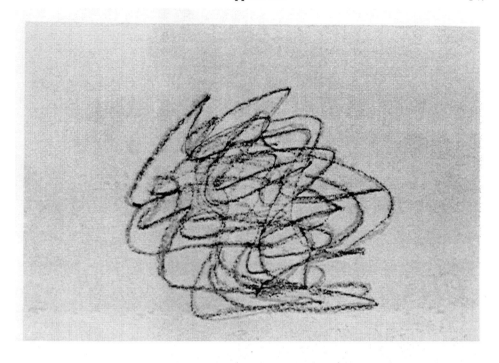

Figure 23. Tasks 3 and 4–A Scribble and a Picture Created from the Scribble: A Tornado (John Franklin).

of John's drawings, which lack interplay and relationships. The omission of interpersonal communication and connection with others appears to be a prevalent theme for him. The characters and situations presented, such as a distant view of the world, a tornado, closed doors, and undifferentiated family members, suggest a possible orientation to crisis or upset, and no support for growth.

Recommendations:

Based upon this assessment and clinical history, the following recommendations are offered:

1. Weekly individual and art therapy to facilitate emotional and cognitive development.
2. Family therapy to clarify and process family issues and to help develop communication between family members.
3. Group and play therapy to help develop socialization skills.
4. Additional psychological testing to rule out neuropsychological problems and learning disabilities.

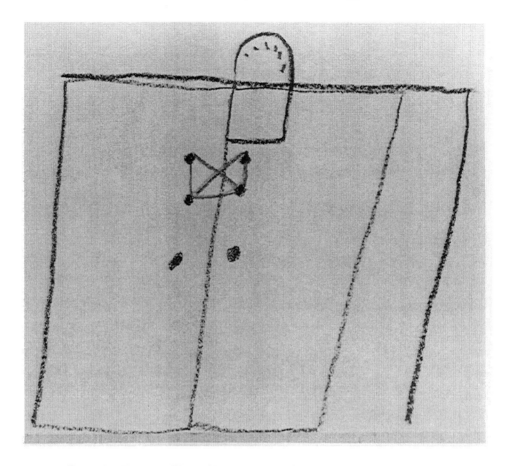

Figure 24. Task 5–A Place of Importance: A Picture Museum (John Franklin).

Clinical Art Therapy Goal and Objectives:

Based on the findings, the following art therapy goal and objectives are proposed for this boy:

ANNUAL GOAL

Through the process of art therapy, the student will demonstrate cognitive growth, better emotional regulation, and amplified adaptive behavior styles conducive to healthy psychosocial adjustment.

OBJECTIVES

The student will:
1. Develop personal expression.

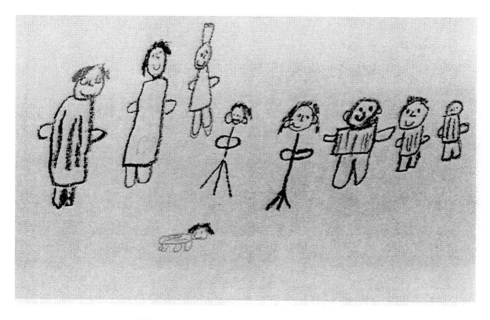

Figure 25. Task 6–John's Family (John Franklin).

2. Channel aggressive impulses.
3. Use artwork to clarify thoughts and feelings.
4. Improve ability to express thoughts and feelings.
5. Experiment with a broader repertoire of adaptive interpersonal behaviors.

APPENDIX D. SAMPLE GOAL AND OBJECTIVES REPORT FOR THE IEP

Art Therapy Program
GOAL AND OBJECTIVES REPORT
for the IEP
1992–1993

STUDENT NAME: <u>John Franklin</u>   DATE OF BIRTH: <u>January 29, 1982</u>

SCHOOL: <u>Children's Development Center</u>   ART THERAPIST: <u>Janet Bush, A.T.R.</u>

Based on the Art Therapy Assessment completed on September 24, 1992 and October 1, 1992, the following art therapy goal and objectives are proposed for the 1992–93 school year.

ANNUAL GOAL

Through the process of Art Therapy, the student will demonstrate cognitive growth, better emotional regulation, and amplified adaptive behavior styles conducive to healthy psychosocial adjustment.

OBJECTIVES

The student will:
1. develop personal expression
2. channel aggressive impulses
3. use artwork to clarify thoughts and feelings
4. improve ability to express thoughts and feelings
5. experiment with a broader repertoire of adaptive interpersonal behaviors

---

APPENDIX E. SAMPLE OF ANNUAL ART THERAPY GOALS AND SHORT–TERM OBJECTIVES

Art Therapy Program
GUIDELINES FOR DEVELOPING ANNUAL ART THERAPY GOALS AND SHORT–TERM OBJECTIVES

These guidelines can assist in program documentation.*

I. Definition of Terms
  A. Goal
    1. Long-Term
      a. Projects the improvement desired.
      b. Specifies the outcome that will be observed if the treatment plan is successful.
      c. Has relatively broad scope and demonstrates long-term changes.
    2. Guidelines
      a. Goals are written from the perspective of the student's behavior.
      b. Goals are written in behavioral terms.
      c. Goals are relevant. They are based on assessment data and are pertinent to the problem.
      d. Goals are useful. They specify the aim or purpose of related service.
      e. Goals are realistic. (1) They are achievable given the student's abilities. (2) They stem logically from the student's present level of functioning and expected length of related service (usually one school year).
  B. Objectives
    1. Short-Term
      a. Are statements of the process relevant to reaching the goal.
      b. Have specific steps that the student will demonstrate toward achieving the goal.
      c. Are narrower in scope than the goal and indicate a specified amount of achievement.
    2. Guidelines
      a. The objectives are observable and result-oriented. They identify steps or increments of behavior the student will exhibit.
      b. The objectives are pertinent.
        (1) Objectives correlate with the assessment data, problem, and goal.
        (2) Objectives reflect changes in assessment data.

---

    c. The objectives are realistic and individualized.
       (1) Objectives are achievable given the student's strengths and abilities.
       (2) Objectives reflect a consideration of the student's developmental level, psychodynamics, and psychopathology.
    d. The objectives set standards. They are used as evaluation criteria. Student behavior is measured against objectives in determining progress toward meeting the goal.
    e. The objectives are useful. They help direct interventions by specifying the aims of the interventions.

II. Format

Writing Goals and Objectives

  1. Order of priority

    The most important is stated first.

  2. Area to improve
    a. Cognitive growth
    b. Emotional regulation
    c. Social behavior
    d. Physical development

  3. How it will improve

    Through the process involved in art therapy.

  4. How much it will improve (degree of change)

    Percentage of time or percentage of opportunities given.
    (The percentage is an estimate based on the student's present level of functioning).

  5. How improvement will be measured (criteria for measuring change)
    a. Formal qualities and content of artwork.
    b. Observations of behavior.
    c. Verbalizations by student.

III. Examples of Documented Goals and Objectives

A list of potential long-term goals and short-term objectives is provided. While this list is lengthy, it is by no means exhaustive. "Individualized" means that the goal or objective is designed to meet the specific needs of the student. However, certain patterns of art therapy objectives do exist, and a compilation of these objectives can be developed. What follows is an overview of a categorization of goals and objectives, cited to assist art therapists in developing their own technique for writing IEP's at their place of employment.

  A. Goals

    1. Some IEP's discuss annual goals without reference to special education programs or related services. However, some annual goals are more service-specific. Below are examples of specific annual art therapy goals.

      a. Cognitive Growth

      Through the process of art therapy the student will demonstrate improved skills in cognitive functioning.

  b. Emotional Regulation
   (1) Through the process of art therapy the student will develop a recognition of, and, consequently, a better regulation of, emotional drives.
   (2) The student will develop a self-image based on feelings of competency and adequacy through participation in art therapy.
  c. Social Behavior
   Through the process of art therapy, the student will experiment with a broader repertoire of adaptive interpersonal behaviors.
  d. Physical Development
   Through the process of art therapy, the student will demonstrate improved integration of sensory-motor systems.

B. Objectives
 1. Cognitive Growth
  a. Expression of Thought
   (1) The student will broaden his cognitive repertoire of intellectual concepts in the form of 50 percent more schema (graphic symbols).
   (2) The student will organize intellectual concepts in graphic form 75 percent of the time.
  b. Flexibility
   (1) The student will strive toward risk-taking ventures during 50 percent of the opportunities given.
   (2) The student will demonstrate skills in spontaneity, yet inhibit impulsiveness 50 percent of the time.
  c. Attending/Focusing
   (1)The student will use art as a means of focusing thoughts and carry through with ideas in a logical, sequential progression 75 percent of the time.
   (2) The student will work with purpose and increase his/her attention span during 75 percent of the opportunities given.
  d. Communication
   The student will improve his/her graphic expression of thoughts and feelings and promote a depth of self-expression through art greater than 50 percent of his/her present level.
 2. Emotional Regulation
  a. Frustration Tolerance/Delayed Gratification
   (1) The student will improve his/her frustration tolerance by evidencing a 50 percent reduction in defeatist attitudes and self-destructive themes in his/her approach to the materials and in the content of the works of art.
   (2) The student will accept delayed gratification as opposed to immediate gratification during 80 percent of the opportunities given.
  b. Self-Monitoring/Evaluating

   (1) The student will improve the frequency of evaluating, redefining, and correcting perceived errors in his/her work by 50 percent of his/her current level.

   (2) The student will develop skills in reflective approaches to his/her artwork as measured by 50 percent improvement over his/her level of functioning.

 c. Control

   (1) The student will acquire 60 percent more impulse control as indicated in choice of art materials and in use of graphic symbols.

   (2) The student will strengthen control over cognitive associative functioning as indicated in graphic representation.

 d. Fantasy vs. Reality/Sublimation/Ego Development

   (1) The student will use art as a means of testing and verifying reality ties during 80 percent of the opportunities given.

   (2) The student will sublimate sexual and aggressive impulses into more appropriate and acceptable channels during 80 percent of the opportunities given.

 e. Release/Express/Work Through Emotions

   (1) The student will reconcile feelings of anger (or stress, frustration, vulnerability, dependency needs, etc.) through the creation of art in an art therapy setting.

   (2) The student will develop more adaptive approaches to the management of apprehension, anxiety, depression, stress, etc., during 50 percent of the opportunities given.

   (3) The student will evidence a 50 percent reduction in aggressive themes in his/her works of art over the course of treatment throughout the school year.

 f. Self-Image

   (1) The student will attempt self-confrontation in terms of feelings related to self-image and concept during 50 percent of the opportunities given.

   (2) The student will achieve a greater sense of security evidenced by a 50 percent reduction in themes illustrating a need for protection in his/her art.

3. Adaptive Behavioral Styles

 a. Independence

   (1) The student will demonstrate skills in assertiveness and independence 50 percent of the time.

   (2) The student will develop skills to evidence a 50 percent increase in making decisions.

 b. Maturation

   (1) The student will develop and demonstrate a more mature posture during 80 percent of the opportunities given as measured by the student's behavior, verbalizations, and works of art.

      (2) The student will demonstrate 50 percent less egocentrism in graphic as well as behavioral portrayal.

      (3) The student will develop skills and resources in the appropriate and successful acquisition of satisfaction from the environment during 75 percent of the opportunities given.

  c. Socialization

      (1) The student will portray 50 percent more interpersonal interaction in his/her works of art.

      (2) The student will develop a therapeutic relationship with the art therapist.

      (3) The student will engage in sharing and group cooperation during 75 percent of the opportunities given in group art therapy.

  d. Positive Peer Interaction

      (1) The student will share his/her art experiences positively with the group 80 percent of the time.

      (2) The student will demonstrate appropriate interaction with peers during 80 percent of the opportunities given.

  e. Group Identity

  The student will develop insight and an accurate perception of his/her behavior through group feedback and art experiences as measured by his/her behavior and content in artistic production.

  f. Motivation/Initiative/Responsibility

      (1) The student will demonstrate motivation to produce works of art and complete 80 percent of the projects self-initiated.

      (2) The student will attend the art therapy group 80 percent of the time.

      (3) The student will work spontaneously and voluntarily with the group 80 percent of the time.

4. Physical Development

  a. Figure-Ground/Parts-to-Whole

      (1) The student will be able to attend to and to differentiate between the figure (symbol) created and the surrounding background in his/her works of art with 75 percent accuracy.

      (2) The student will be able to create schema (graphic symbols) based on a collection of integrated parts (appropriately placed) during 75 percent of the opportunities given.

      (3) The student will evidence 50 percent less overlapping of schema on a single background.

  b. Directionality

  The student will demonstrate improved discrimination between left and right directions in space during 75 percent of the opportunities given in the creation of three-dimensional works of art.

  c. Sequencing

The student will complete a sophisticated project, following the appropriate sequential progression during 75 percent of the opportunities given.

c. Fine-Motor Coordination

The student will show 50 percent improvement in eye-hand coordination demonstrated by his/her approach to the materials (such as by accurately outlining and filling space in color, by improved precision in cutting with scissors, and by improved precision in applying paint to paper with a paint brush).

APPENDIX F. SAMPLE PROGRESS REPORT

Art Therapy Program
PROGRESS REPORT

STUDENT NAME: __John Franklin__   SCHOOL: __Children's Development Center__

DATE OF BIRTH: __1/29/82__   DATE: __5/27/93__

ART THERAPIST: __Janet Bush, A.T.R.__

John Franklin has been in individualized art therapy during the 1992–93 school year. Goals have included helping him to identify and deal with unresolved issues, such as handling anger and working through the losses in his life.

John enjoys art therapy, and uses art materials and processes creatively. He is compliant and easily directed to participate in projects. However, John is unusually nonverbal when sessions focus on encouraging him to share personal background information and feelings.

John recognizes that he has problems handling anger. This year he worked on a book describing some of his inappropriate behaviors. However, many unresolved emotional/developmental issues remain in John's background, which continually cause him emotional distress. The most important issue is the loss of his biological parents.

In a recent session, John drew a picture (see Figure 26) for one of the tasks on the Levick Emotional and Cognitive Art Therapy Assessment (LECATA). The drawing, entitled "The Haunted House," was described by John as "a place where ghosts lived." He had difficulty tying the picture to a story or making any kind of association between it and something else, although it is suspected that many of John's issues, relating to nurturance, security, and safety, may be correlated with this drawing.

When compared with his October 1991 assessment drawing, on which he scored below the norm for his age, this drawing reflected a similar score, indicating that cognitively and emotionally, John has made little progress in his development. This drawing shows that he continues to use immature defenses: isolation of affect, denial, imitation, and isolation, all of which are atypical for John's age group. Cognitively, his forms reflect a lack of sophistication and detail that indicate he has not advanced intellectually to the level normally observed in youngsters his age.

John continues to need help in processing the traumatic losses in his life and in learning how to assert his anger in a healthy and productive way. It is recommended that art therapy continue for the next school year to assist him in reaching his academic and emotional potential.

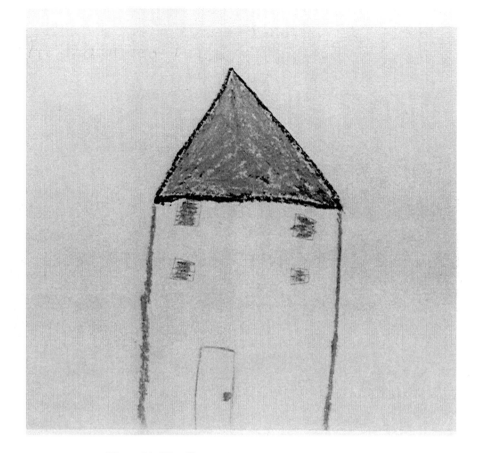

Figure 26. The Haunted House (John Franklin).

APPENDIX G. SAMPLE ART THERAPY REPORT FOR CASE CONFERENCE

Art Therapy Program
REPORT FOR CASE CONFERENCE

STUDENT NAME: _____ DATE OF BIRTH: _____

GRADE: _____ SCHOOL: _____

REPORT DATE: _____ ART THERAPIST: _____

  A. *Levels of Functioning*
     1. Emotional _____ 2. Cognitive _____ 3. Developmental Score _____
  B. *Observations*
     1. Behavioral observations
     2. Significant characteristics
     3. Impulse control, frustration tolerance, attention span, affect, verbal expression, cooperative effort, risk taking, ability to engage
  C. *Clinical Impressions Derived from Artwork*
     1. Defense mechanisms and how employed
     2. Symbolic imagery and suggested themes/issues
     3. Strengths/weaknesses
  D. *Recommendations*
     1. Suggested treatment focus
     2. Implications for other settings

APPENDIX H. SAMPLE SCHEDULE

Art Therapy Program
SCHEDULE

School Year: 1996-1997

Art Therapist: Jane Kelly, A.T.R.-BC

Monday (RM 16)		Tuesday (RM 15)		Wednesday (RM 16)		Thursday (RM 15)		Friday (RM 16)	
School: Palm Elem.		School: Lanier Elem.		School: Palm Elem.		School: Lanier Elem.		School: Palm Elem.	
8:15 - 8:45	Set up	8:15 - 8:45	Set up	8:15 - 8:45	Set up	8:15-8:45	Set up	8:15-8:45	Set up
8:45 - 9:15	Individual	8:45 - 9:30	Group	8:45 - 9:15	Individual	8:45-9:15	Individual	8:45-9:15	Individual
9:30 -10:15	Individual	9:40 -10:15	Individual	9:20-10:50	Iindividual	9:20-10:05	Dyad	9:20-10:15	Group
10:30-11:30	Dyad	10:15-10:45	Individual	10:50-11:45	Group	10:10-10:40	Individual	10:20-11:30	Assessment
11:30-12:00	LUNCH	10:50-11:30	Dyad	11:45-12:15	LUNCH	10:45-11:15	Individual	11:30-12:00	LUNCH
12:15- 1:00	Group	11:30-12:00	Individual	12:15-12:45	Documentation	11:20-12:00	Individual	12:00-1:00	Documentation
1:00- 1:30	Individual	12:00-12:30	Meeting with Clinicians/Planning	12:45- 1:20	Travel to Meeting	12:00-12:30	LUNCH	1:15-1:50	Individual
1:30- 2:30	Meeting with Clinicians/ Planning	12:30- 1:00	LUNCH	1:30- 3:15	Staff Development/Department Meeting	12:30-1:00	Individual	1:50-2:30	Group
1:30- 2:30	Documentation	1:00- 2:00	Assessment			1:00 - 1:30	Individual	2:30-3:15	Meeting w/ Teachers
2:30- 3:15	Case Conference	2:00- 3:15	Documentation			1:30 - 2:00	Individual		
						2:00 - 2:30	Meeting w/ Teachers		
						2:30 - 3:15	Case Conference		

THIS SCHEDULE IS CURRENT AS OF THIS DATE: September 16, 1996

APPENDIX I. SAMPLE SESSION TREATMENT PLAN

Art Therapy Program
SESSION TREATMENT PLAN

Student: <u>John Franklin</u>   DATE OF BIRTH: <u>1/29/82</u>   SESSION DATE: <u>5/25/92</u>

LONG-TERM GOAL
Through the process of art therapy, the student will demonstrate cognitive growth, better emotional regulation, and amplified adaptive behavior styles conducive to healthy psychosocial behavior.

SHORT-TERM OBJECTIVE
The student will: (check those that apply) ___ 1. Develop personal expression. ___ 2. Channel aggressive impulses. ___ 3. Use artwork to clarify thoughts and feelings. ___ 4. Improve ability to express thoughts and feelings. ___ 5. Experiment with a broader repertoire of adaptive interpersonal behaviors.

PROCEDURE
The development of the student's self-concept and his feelings of mastery and control over his environment will be facilitated through his free-choice activity. The student will be encouraged to discuss his thoughts and feelings in relation to the project he has selected.

MATERIALS
Free choice

EVALUATION OF SESSION
John selected oil clay and created an image of a robot. He associated the robot with television shows and commented that he spends much time watching television. His thoughts and feelings related to his free time were explored.

FOLLOW UP
Continue with John's lead to create spontaneous works of art.

APPENDIX J. SAMPLE PROGRAM SUPPORT CHECKLIST

Art Therapy Program
PROGRAM SUPPORT CHECKLIST

NAME OF ART THERAPIST: _____ SCHOOL: _____

NAME OF STUDENT: _____ EXCEPTIONALITY: _____

ART THERAPY EXPERIENCE: _____

OBSERVER: _____ DATE: _____

Key: ✓ acceptable   *needs improvement

STRATEGIES OF ART THERAPIST

___ Assembles materials prior to activity.

Implements art therapy objectives through the following steps:

___ Sets time limit before work session begins and reiterates time limit during session (if necessary)
___ Introduces materials and concepts
___ Demonstrates (if necessary)
___ Distributes materials
___ Provides guidance
___ Shows an understanding of student's artwork and behavior
___ Uses appropriate intervention skills
___ Encourages cooperative care of materials and cleanup
___ Engages in evaluation and closure

THERAPEUTIC ALLIANCE WITH STUDENT

___ Relates to student with respect and empathy
___ Shows a concerned and caring attitude toward student
___ Gives student individual attention
___ Leads student to use appropriate behavior
___ Encourages student to explore thoughts and feelings
___ Does not criticize student
___ Helps student feel accepted even when proscribing certain behaviors

PHYSICAL CONDITIONS

Arranges compatible environment through:

___ space   ___ materials
___ furnishings   ___ organization
___ equipment   ___ accessibility

DOCUMENTATION PROCEDURES

Follows record-keeping procedures:
__ Maintains record of development in the form of session treatment plans
__ Maintains record of development of art products
__ Completes Art Therapy Assessment Reports
__ Completes Goal and Objectives on IEP
__ Completes Student Progress Reports
__ Completes Staff Development Session Documentation
__ Maintains Parent Permission Consent Forms

OTHER

__ Participates in student placement meetings
__ Participates in family meetings
__ Communicates with school personnel
__ Provides art therapy staff development programs
__ Follows administrative requirements of the school
__ Participates in Art Therapy Department meetings
__ Carries out activities of the Art Therapy Department

NOTES AND RECOMMENDATIONS

_____
_____
_____
_____
_____
_____
_____
_____
_____
_____
_____
_____
_____

APPENDIX K. SAMPLE LETTER REQUESTING
MEDIA COVERAGE

Art Therapy Program
LETTER REQUESTING MEDIA COVERAGE

March 1, 1994

Mr. John Mason, Editor
Community News
1450 Prairie Drive
Miami, FL 33124

Dear Mr. Mason:

Art therapy is a dynamic, expanding area of service for people with special needs. Our school district has, over the past fifteen years, developed an innovative and effective Art Therapy Program, and we would like to acquaint the public with some of the ways in which art therapy works. Would you consider preparing a written article about the art therapy process? We can present some actual scenes of how an individual session might be conducted, and can use original artwork and slides to elaborate the process.

I look forward to a favorable reply, and can be contacted at 995-1889. I am enclosing a background statement and visual sequence example of a progressive art therapy experience.

Sincerely,

Janet Bush, A.T.R.

JB:syg

Enclosure

APPENDIX L. SAMPLE PRESS RELEASE

Art Therapy Program

ART THERAPY IS HELPING TO PAINT A BRIGHTER FUTURE FOR MIAMI'S TEACHERS AND STUDENTS AFFECTED BY HURRICANE ANDREW

Artwork can reveal a great deal to the Art Therapist about an individual's state of mind. In the Miami schools, Art Therapy is both diagnostic and therapeutic. It creates a conduit through which trained art therapists can help individuals to talk about their private demons.

Teachers and students in Miami's schools have been getting a chance to picture their feelings about Hurricane Andrew with help from the Art Therapy Department. As part of a crisis response effort, the art therapists are working in selected schools to help individuals cope with the hurricane aftermath. The effort is designed to help them deal with their reactions to the experience. Students and staff are encouraged to "draw out" the fears and anxieties they connect with the hurricane.

A number of questions are asked; such as, What are the signs and symbols that reveal what people are dealing with? How can art production assist people through a crisis?

Art therapy is an approach to understanding that does not depend on words. Through art therapy, individuals are helped to expand their understanding, to grow, to cope, and to improve their lives. We would like to show you how it works.

**Photo Opportunities

Contact: Janet Bush, 995-1889.

APPENDIX M. SAMPLE CONSENT FORMS 1, 2, AND 3

Art Therapy Program
CONSENT FORMS*

1. Documenting a Case Study

Authorization Form

I, the undersigned parent or legal guardian, do hereby give my consent for my child, _____, to be the subject of a paper presented at the American Art Therapy Association Conference on _____.

(Date)

I understand that my child's name will remain anonymous, a pseudonym will be assigned, and he/she will be identified by sex, age, and other selected information relevant in providing a case history. No formal family background information will be described to identify the family in any way. Slides of my child's artwork will be presented at the conference, and a paper with accompanying artwork may appear in the Proceedings of the conference (a published document), or other journal.

_____ _____
Date   Signature of Parent or Legal Guardian

2. Authorization to Exhibit Art

I, the undersigned parent or legal guardian, do hereby give my consent and authorize the exhibition of my child's, _____'s, artwork, described as: _____ on the following date: _____, subject only to the condition that he/she will not be identified by name on any art objects. I understand this exhibition may be used for inservice presentations, case conferences, or other educational research purposes at the school.

_____ _____
Date   Signature of Parent or Legal Guardian

3. Photographing Art Work

I, the undersigned parent or legal guardian, do hereby give my consent and authorize the photographing of my child's, _____'s, artworks, subject only to the condition that he/she will not be identified by name on any art objects, slides, or photographs thereof. I understand these photographs or slides may be used for inservice presentations, case conferences, or other educational or research purposes at the school.

_____ _____
Date   Signature of Parent or Legal Guardian

*All Rights reserved. Reprinted with permission from the American Art Therapy Association, Resource Packet for Art Therapists in the Schools, 1984.

166

APPENDIX N. SAMPLE SCHOOL ART THERAPY JOB SPECIFICATIONS

Art Therapy Program
SCHOOL ART THERAPY JOB SPECIFICATIONS

POSITION TITLE: School Art Therapist

SUMMARY OF POSITION

Art therapy is designed to meet the individually assessed special needs of students. In addition to direct work with regular students, art therapists present inservice programs for teachers, school support personnel, and administrators, and provide art therapy assessments and diagnostic work and treatment for special students who are explicitly referred from a variety of school programs.

RATIONALE

Art therapy services are designed to assist the student in benefiting from education by enhancing the student's potential for learning. Art therapy can facilitate appropriate social behavior and can promote healthy affective development so that the student can be more receptive to academic involvement and can realize social and academic potential.

SPECIALIZED DUTIES OF ART THERAPISTS

Art therapists are responsible for evaluating, planning, and implementing treatment programs for individual students and for small groups of students according to the principles and practices of art therapy.

QUALIFICATIONS

Art therapists are professionals with a master's degree in art therapy from an accredited program in art therapy, and who are either in the process of obtaining professional registration from the Art Therapy Credentials Board or who have already received professional registration from the Art Therapy Credentials Board.

NEED BY ART THERAPISTS IN SCHOOLS TO OBTAIN STATE TEACHING CERTIFICATES

Art therapists do not teach courses, but the American Art Therapy Association believes that a credentialed art therapist meets criteria equivalent to criteria for teaching certification in a specialized area of education. Notwithstanding, many states require these professionals to obtain teaching credentials to work in schools. In those states, certification should be considered in any educational area.

SALARY REQUIREMENTS

Salaries for art therapists in schools should be commensurate with those for other professionals in schools; that is, teachers, administrators, and psychologists.

CASELOAD

The art therapist/student ratio is based upon the individual needs of the students and the resources available. The number of individual and group art therapy sessions scheduled a week, in addition to assessment/intake time, should limit the number of students seen to no more than 20–25 a week.

STUDENTS WHO SHOULD RECEIVE ART THERAPY SERVICES

Art therapy is valuable for all students, but especially for the disabled—those experiencing difficulty in school because of personal crisis, and for those in alternative settings. Art therapy offers a therapeutic/diagnostic/prescriptive approach to the students who have been identified as disabled and to the other students with special needs.

SCHEDULING

Although one art therapist per 20–25 students is the recommended maximum caseload, this ratio may vary depending upon:

1. Type of art therapy service provided
   a. art therapy assessment
   b. individual sessions
   c. small group sessions
   d. consultation services
2. Length of art therapy sessions
   a. 60 minutes for assessment procedure
   b. 30 to 60 minutes per individual
   c. 45 to 60 minutes per small group
3. Length of professional day
   a. full-time employee
   b. part-time employee
   c. part-time consultant
4. Available facilities
   a. separate art therapy room fully equipped
   b. no designated art therapy room
5. Scheduling factors
   a. student's individualized schedule
   b. related service providers' schedules
   c. art therapist's schedule
6. Age and developmental level of student
   a. cognitive functioning
   b. emotional functioning and general level of personality development
   c. level of physical maturity and functioning
   d. social behavior
   e. academic functioning

RESPONSIBILITIES

- **Establish a Therapeutic Environment**

  Maintain a physically safe environment for conducting art therapy (i.e., adhere to health and safety regulations, ensure proper ventilation and storage of materials, monitor use of sharp items, maintain universal precautions regarding health hazards.

Create and maintain a therapeutic environment that is psychologically safe (i.e., provide structure and behavioral management, ensure privacy and confidentiality).

Design a therapeutic environment conducive to making art (e.g., create an inviting atmosphere with a variety of accessible materials).

Establish a relationship with the student through art expression and verbal interaction.

- **Implement Student Assessment Procedures**

Discuss or otherwise establish a reason for referral with a referral source.

Orient the student to the therapeutic process in general and art therapy in particular.

Obtain demographic information (e.g., age, family status), history (e.g., events precipitating current contact with therapist and medical, developmental, psychosocial, and psychiatric histories), and information on current level of functioning and mental status.

Evaluate the likelihood that the student will do harm to himself/herself or to others in the immediate future.

Discuss assessment procedures with the student.

Select assessment techniques, which may include art, verbal tasks, and written tasks.

Conduct the art therapy assessment.

Evaluate the art products and process, and other data derived from the assessment to identify student's strengths and needs.

Document assessment results, including art therapy goals and short-term objectives, within an appropriate time frame.

Review records from other professionals (e.g., psychiatrist, school psychologist), as needed.

Evaluate appropriateness of art therapy as a treatment modality for the student.

Refer the student for further evaluation by other professionals (e.g., physician, psychiatrist, psychologist).

- **Plan Treatment**

Formulate the art therapy treatment plan.

Discuss the goals with the student.

Recommend and follow up on treatment by other professionals (e.g., physician, psychiatrist, psychologist), if appropriate.

Discuss the school art therapy treatment plan with school professionals involved in student's treatment.

- **Implement Treatment Plans**

  Schedule art therapy sessions for individuals or groups of students.

  Structure the art therapy milieu for effective treatment.

  Provide an art therapy treatment program according to the goals and objectives outlined in the art therapy assessment.

  Obtain equipment and materials necessary to maintain an inventory that allows flexibility of expression.

  Select art materials and processes.

  Adapt the art materials and processes to the needs of specific populations.

  Prepare the art materials to be used in the therapy session.

  Discuss ground rules for art therapy sessions (e.g., use of materials, behavior in the therapeutic environment) with the student.

  Instruct the student in the use of art media.

  Make a note of and draw inferences from student's art product, affect, behavior, commentary, and interaction with group members (if any) during the art-making process.

  Use art processes to facilitate expression and exploration of feelings, thoughts, perceptions, and other relevant clinical material.

  Use art therapy processes to give feedback, increase self-perception, enhance self-worth, develop ego strength, and promote growth and healing.

  Promote the creation of art through the use of art therapy processes.

  Use verbal interactions, when appropriate, to promote mutual understanding of student's art processes and products.

  Facilitate group processes in ways appropriate to the student's needs.

  Maintain an appropriate pace for therapy, based on the student's strengths and needs and the therapeutic goals.

  Evaluate the student's progress toward therapeutic goals on a regular basis.

  Modify the treatment plan and therapeutic goals, as necessary, throughout the course of therapy.

  Determine whether the display of student artwork in sessions and public forums would be appropriate.

  Communicate regularly with other professionals involved in the student's treatment.

  Provide consultation with other professionals on specific cases and art therapy processes.

  Facilitate the termination process in ways appropriate to student needs or circumstances.

Refer the student to another credentialed art therapist or mental health professional if appropriate.

- **Maintain Documentation**

  Maintain a record of student attendance.

  Maintain records of each art therapy session, including the process and content of artwork, verbalizations, and behavior.

  Submit required reports on a monthly, quarterly, and annual basis, as may be specified by the school program.

  If necessary, photograph student's artwork as specified, maintaining confidentiality of student's identity, and acquiring permission from parents.

  Submit and share written assessment results, individualized treatment plans, progress notes, and annual narrative reports according to school procedures.

  Document the initial assessment, the art therapy treatment plan, and the student's progress in therapy.

  Maintain appropriate documentation and labeling of the student's artwork, including student's name, medium, content, and date of creation.

  Prepare written reports, as needed, for agencies and institutions (e.g., courts, youth and family service agencies) and for professionals involved in the student's treatment.

  Maintain a file of appropriate consent and release forms for use with student artwork.

- **Provide Ongoing Communication with School Personnel**

  Participate in interdisciplinary staff meetings.

  Consult with classroom teachers, psychologists, and other related service providers regarding case management.

  Consult with student's parents or legal guardian, and transmit the information to appropriate school staff.

- **Maintain an Appropriate Physical Facility**

  Follow the safety requirements of the school.

  Demonstrate proper purchase, use, handling, and maintenance of art therapy supplies and equipment to insure the cost effectiveness of the program.

  a. Purchase supplies and equipment that conform to the standards of safety established by the school and art therapy program.

  b. Insure proper storage, maintenance, and handling of toxic, flammable, and otherwise dangerous art supplies.

  c. Insure the proper use, handling, and maintenance of such art equipment as a kiln and paper cutter.

Report defective supplies and equipment, and remove such items from circulation for repair or disposal.

- **Engage in Professional Development**

  Represent the art therapy program and art therapy department at professional meetings and conferences.

  Clarify the theory and practice of art therapy for the administration, teaching faculty, multidisciplinary related service providers, parents, and students. Present theoretical and practical aspects of art therapy to outside professional and lay groups through professional development programs.

- **Maintain Professionalism and Ethics**

  Promote a professional atmosphere in the department and maintain a professional demeanor.

  Provide art therapy services in accordance with the AATA Code of Ethics for Art Therapists, the AATA General Standards of Practice Document, and the policies and procedures of the school district in which services are provided.

  Provide art therapy services that are appropriate to your role as primary or adjunctive therapist.

  Preserve student images (originals and copies) in a secure and confidential manner.

  Conduct self-appraisal of art therapy services provided to students on an ongoing basis.

  Recognize professional and personal limitations in providing effective art therapy services (e.g., biases, specialty areas, physical and psychological factors that affect the therapist).

  Consult with, and seek supervision from, credentialed professionals, and review literature as needed, to provide appropriate and effective art therapy services.

  Develop and maintain contact with a network of professionals who may provide specialized art therapy or other therapeutic services to students (e.g., treatment team).

  Maintain knowledge of and inform students and families about community resources (e.g., leisure activities, education, social services).

  Educate lay persons and professionals on the profession and practice of art therapy.

  Conduct inservice training for art therapists and other mental health professionals.

  Present and offer professional services in an appropriate manner.

  Engage in making art.

  Provide art therapy services in compliance with federal, state, and local regulations regarding business practices, the provision of mental health services, and related issues (e.g., Americans with Disabilities Act).

Abide by state and local laws regarding the reporting of physical/sexual abuse and neglect.

Recognize and adhere to student rights and entitlements.

Respect the student's right to confidentiality.

Maintain art therapy credentials with the Art Therapy Credentials Board.

Promote and engage in continuing educational endeavors.

Represent the art therapy program favorably to the school and community.

Maintain your availability to other staff members as a resource person.

Engage in professional research endeavors in the promotion of art therapy.

BIBLIOGRAPHY

Ahrentzen, S., Jue, G., Skorpanich, M., and Evans, G. (1982). School environments and stress. In G.W. Evans (Ed.), *Environmental stress* (pp. 225–255). Cambridge, Eng.: University Press.

American Art Therapy Association, Inc. (1986). *Resource packet for art therapists in schools*. Mundelein, IL: Author.

American Art Therapy Association, Inc. (1994). *Ethical standards for art therapists*. Mundelein, IL: Author.

Anderson, F.E. (1978). *Art for all the children: A creative source book for the impaired child*. Springfield, IL: Charles C Thomas.

Anderson, F.E. (1992). *Art for all the children: Approaches to art therapy for children with disabilities*. (2nd ed.). Springfield, IL: Charles C Thomas.

Art in the Lives of Persons with Special Needs. *Proceedings of a joint conference of the National Art Education Association, Inc., and the American Art Therapy Association, Inc.,* through support of the National Committee Arts for the Handicapped, August 7–8, 1980. NCAH, J. F. Kennedy Center for the Performing Arts, Education Office, Washington, D.C. 20566.

Art Therapy Credentials Board, Inc. (1993). *Adopted revised standards and procedures for registration*. Mundelein, IL: Author.

Art Therapy in the Schools (1985). A position paper in the resource packet for art therapists in schools. Mundelein, IL. American Art Therapy Association.

Bettleheim, B. (1974). *A Home for the Heart*. New York: Knopf.

Brophy, J. (1983). Classroom organization and management. *The Elementary School Journal,* 84(4), 265–85.

Bush, J. (1976). *Art therapy: Its use in effecting change in school-age children with acute learning problems*. Unpublished thesis prepared at the Hahnemann Medical University, Philadelphia, PA.

Bush, J. (1979). *A pilot art education therapy program*. Dade County Public Schools. Miami, FL.

Bush, J. (1980). *A report on the pilot art education therapy program*. Dade County Public Schools, Miami, FL.

Bush, J. *Conference proceedings: Visual arts education and the mainstreamed exceptional student*. May 3, 1980.

Bush, J. (1980). *Response to a not so special approach to art programming for the person with special needs*. Study conference of the American Art Therapy Association and National Art Education Association, August 7–8, 1980. Reston, VA.

Bush, J. (1981). *Art blends*. Dade County Public Schools. Miami, FL.

Bush, J. (1990). *Art therapy has healing power.* (Publicity packet.) Available from the Dade County Public Schools Art Therapy Program, Division of Exceptional Student Education, Miami, FL.

Bush, J. (1993). *Art therapy program handbook.* Dade County Public Schools, Miami, FL.

Bush, J. (1993). *Draft of standards in school art therapy.* Miami, FL.

Bush, J. (1994). My visualization for 21st century art therapy. *Art Therapy,* 11, 31–32.

Bush, J. (1995). *Art therapy program procedures handbook.* Dade County Public Schools. Miami, FL.

Bush, J. (1995). *Innovate or evaporate: Developing your public relations and marketing innovation quotient.* Dade County Public Schools, Miami, FL.

Cane, F. (1951). *The artist in each of us.* Craftsbury Common, VT: Art Therapy Publications.

Code of Federal Regulations, Parts 100–149 (Revised as of October 1, 1978). Published by the Office of the Federal Register, National Archives and Records Service. Washington, D.C.

Cohen, F. (1974). Introducing art therapy into a school system: Some problems. *Art Psychotherapy* 2:121–136.

Cole, N. (1941). *The arts in the classroom.* New York: John Day.

Dade County Public Schools (1978). *CurriculArt—An art education curriculum.* Miami, Florida: Author.

Dade County Public Schools. (1979, 1985). Office of Educational Accountability. Miami, Florida: Author.

Dinkmeyer, D., Dinkmeyer, D., Jr., and Sperry, L. (1987). Alderian counseling and psychotherapy, 2nd ed. Columbus, OH: Merrill.

Eastern Virginia Medical School (1994). *Course catalog.* Norfolk, VA: Author

Fischer, M.A. et al. (1978). Spontaneous art: A program designed for the individual child in the primary and secondary school setting. In: Mandel, B., Shoemaker, R., and Hays, R. (Eds.). *The Dynamics of Creativity.* Proceedings of the Eighth Annual Conference, American Art Therapy Association, Baltimore, MD.

Individualized Education Program/IEP (1989). Tallahassee, FL, State of Florida Department of Education, Division of Public Schools, Bureau of Education of Exceptional Students.

Legislative Alliance of Creative Arts Therapies. *Testimony regarding PL 94-142 Proposed Regulatory Changes, 1982.* Washington, D.C.: U.S. Department of Education.

Levick, M.F. (1978). *Quality in training.* Paper presented at the American Art Therapy Association Conference. Los Angeles, CA.

Levick, M. F. et al (1989). *The Levick Emotional and Cognitive Art Therapy Assessment.* (available from Myra Levick, 19730 Dinner Key Dr., Boca Raton, Florida 33498).

Levick, M. F. (1989). Reflections: On the road to educating the creative arts therapist. *The Arts in Psychotherapy.* 16, 57–60.

Levick, M. F. (1994). To be or not to be. *Art Therapy.* 11. (2), 97–100.

Lowenfeld, V., and Brittain, W.L. (1957). *Creative and mental growth.* (3rd ed.). New York: MacMillan.

Lowenfeld, V., and Brittain, W. L. (1970). *Creative and mental growth* (4th ed.). New York: MacMillan.

Lowenfeld, V., and Brittain, W. L. (1975). *Creative and mental growth* (5th ed.). New York: MacMillan.

Lowenfeld, V., and Brittain, W. L. (1987). *Creative and mental growth* (8th ed.). New York: MacMillan.

Malchiodi, C. (1987). Art therapy funding from arts-related sources. *American Journal of Art Therapy, 25*, 91–94.

Minar, V., (1978). Report on a pilot study: Art therapy in public schools. In Shoemaker, R., and Gonick-Barris, S., 1978. *The Dynamics of Creativity.* Proceedings of the Seventh Annual Conference. American Art Therapy Association, Baltimore, MD.

Morreau, L., and Anderson, F.E. (1984). Art and the individualized education program. Benefit or burden? *Art Education.* 32(6), 10–14.

Naisbitt, J. and Aburdene, P. (1990). *Megatrends 2000: Ten New Directions for the 1990's.* New York: William Morrow.

National Alliance of Pupil Service Organizations. *Testimony regarding PL 94-142 Proposed Regulatory Changes, September 9, 1982.* Washington, D.C.: U.S. Department of Education.

National Art Education Association (1975). *Art Education.* 28(8), (entire issue).

Pine, S. (1974). Fostering growth through art education, art therapy, and art in psychotherapy. *Art Therapy in Theory and Practice.* Eleanor Ulman, Ed., 60–95. New York: Schocken Books.

Public Law 94-142. (1975). *Education for All Handicapped Children Act.*

Public Law 101-476. (1990). *Individuals with Disabilities Education Act (IDEA).*

Quinn, T., and Hanks, C. (Eds.) (1977). *Coming to our senses: The significance of the arts for american education: A panel report.* J.D. Rockefeller, Jr., Chairman, The Arts Education and Americans Panel. New York: McGraw-Hill.

Robertson, S. (1963). *Rosegarden and labyrinth.* London: Routledge and Kegan Paul.

Stoner, S. D., 1978. Art Education and art therapy: Dynamic duo? In Mandel, B., Shoemaker, R., and Hays, R. (Eds.) *The Dynamics of Creativity. Proceedings of the Eighth Annual Conference,* American Art Therapy Association, Baltimore, MD.

Ursuline College (1994). *Course catalog.* Pepper Pike, OH: Author.

INDEX

179